ESB

D0805256

Duathlon Training and Racing for Ordinary Mortals®

Also by **Steven Jonas, MD, MPH**

The Essential Triathlete: An Introduction to the World of Triathlon

Triathloning for Ordinary Mortals: And Doing the Duathlon Too

101 Ideas and Insights for Triathletes and Duathletes

Championship Triathlon Training, co-authored with George Dallam

Duathlon Training and Racing for **Ordinary Mortals**®: Getting Started and Staying With It

Steven Jonas, MD, MPH

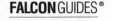

GUILFORD, CONNECTICUT
HELENA, MONTANA
AN IMPRINT OF GLOBE PEQUOT PRESS

To buy books in quantity for corporate use
or incentives, call **(800) 962-0973**
or e-mail **premiums@GlobePequot.com.**

FALCONGUIDES®

Copyright © 2012 by Steven Jonas

ALL RIGHTS RESERVED. No part of this book may be reproduced or transmitted in any
form by any means, electronic or mechanical, including photocopying and recording, or
by any information storage and retrieval system, except as may be expressly permitted in
writing from the publisher. Requests for permission should be addressed to Globe Pequot
Press, Attn: Rights and Permissions Department, P.O. Box 480, Guilford, CT 06437.

FalconGuides is an imprint of Globe Pequot Press.
Falcon, FalconGuides, and Outfit Your Mind are registered trademarks of Morris Book
Publishing , LLC.

Designer: Sheryl P. Kober
Layout artist: Kirsten Livingston
Project editor: Ellen Urban

Library of Congress Cataloging-in-Publication Data is available on file.

ISBN 978-0-7627-7824-9

Printed in the United States of America

10 9 8 7 6 5 4 3 2 1

Portions of the history section in chapter 1 and the original text for chapter 2 were
provided by USA Triathlon and are used with permission. Elements of the text that
previously appeared in Dr. Jonas's columns in the *American Medical Athletic Association
Journal*, *USA Triathlon Magazine*, *101 Ideas and Insights for Triathletes and Duathletes*, and
ACSM's Exercise Is Medicine are also used with permission.

Jeff Matlow's Tao of Triathlon appeared in the Spring 2011 issue of *USAT Magazine*, and is
used with his permission and that of his editor, Jayme Ramson, in chapter 11 of this book.

Medical Disclaimer: The programs in this book are designed for athletes with a
healthy-to-high level of fitness or the physiology to attain a healthy-to-high level of
fitness. Readers should consult a physician before beginning any of the programs
or workouts suggested. If you experience any pain or difficulty with these activities,
stop and consult a healthcare provider.

For my darling wife, Chezna, who has been with me since my one hundredth race. Now and forever.

Contents

Foreword

Duathlon Training and Racing for Ordinary Mortals® is a no-nonsense, concise, and comprehensive book devoted to a sport whose recognition is long overdue.

I have known Steve since 1984, when he competed in the first duathlon that was organized by the New York Triathlon Club, in Brooklyn, New York. Back then we had no idea that twenty-seven years later we would try to remember dates, events, and names from what we now know were the fledgling years of a sport that now attracts mass participation. Since those early days, Steve has competed in over one hundred triathlons and duathlons organized by the New York Triathlon Club as well as over a hundred other local, regional, national, and international events. His unparalleled racing achievements and vast experience are the source for a refreshing, insightful book that deals with every aspect of duathlon, from physical and mental health to competitive success.

As an author of one of the first books written on the subject of triathlon training (*How to Swim, Bike and Run Better*, 1985), I have witnessed how training and racing books have become so scientific and technical that they are hard to comprehend and miss what is perhaps the most critical point of any training guide: to supply information in an accessible, inspirational context. Steve's book, on the other hand, combines technical information with his own real-world experience, and provides the stirring example of an athlete who endures, succeeds, excites, motivates, and exemplifies dedicated, athletic prowess. Through his new book, Steve informs readers of all skill levels that enthusiasm and experience are truly the best teachers.

Steve's book is a treasure trove of his considerable knowledge and experience as a multisport athlete. Readers can trust that Steve's guide provides the best kind of information; his is an approach that is informed by his considerable credentials as a professor of preventive medicine at Stony Brook University's School of Medicine, as a seasoned author of over fifteen books on health and fitness, and, most important, as an international multisport competitor for nearly thirty years.

To the novice, the idea of competing in a duathlon can seem intimidating without proper mental and physical preparation. How often should I train? How hard should I train? What equipment do I need? How can I prevent injuries? These basic questions and related subjects can confound newcomers to the sport and tempt many to give up before they even start. Steve's book provides answers for these aspiring athletes and provides a sourcebook for those who just want a one-stop review of all aspects of recreational and competitive duathlon racing.

There is no better "coach" than Steve since his book easily transfers his duathlon proficiency to his readers; more importantly, Steve imbues his books with his own personal mark—the unmatched joy he derives from duathlon. Not only does Steve share his experience, but he also shares his infectious love for the sport of duathlon and the joy it manifests for him.

As neophytes in any sport, we often feel a sense of detachment when we read training and racing books written by the pros. Steve's book, written by a middle-of-the-pack competitor, is so much easier for the "ordinary mortal" to relate to. Steve's experience as a noted educator and health expert contributes mightily to ease of understanding of his engaging, motivational prose.

Admittedly a slow competitor, Steve can always be counted on to cross the finish line. After reading *Duathlon Training and Racing for Ordinary Mortals®*, readers will have the tools to develop and then personally fine tune the skills that they will need to compete in and derive enjoyment from duathlon.

Unique to this book is a comprehensive assessment of the state of the sport of duathlon as well as a unique and personal history of Steve's singular experience since the first days of the sport. I have watched Steve's personal evolution alongside the development of the sport of duathlon; his unique commitment to multisport competition and his sheer delight in every race he does are dazzling.

I highly recommend this book to anyone from the first-time to the most-experienced duathlete.

Daniel Honig
Founder/President
New York Triathlon Club

Preface

Welcome to the wonderful world of duathlon, a three-segment, two-sport racing event in which you first do a run, then a bike, and finally another run. What? A multisport racing event without swimming? Yes indeed, there is such a thing, and it is this race that this book is all about. Of course there is triathlon, the swim-bike-run event that has dominated multisport racing since it was first developed back in the 1970s. You may well have thought about getting into it, but oh, the thought of swimming just didn't appeal to you. You don't swim, or don't like to swim, or do like it, but have no good place to train, or think that you might be uncomfortable in open water. Or maybe you are indeed a triathlete but want to experience a different approach to multisport racing. Or perhaps you would like a way to ease into it without committing to the technically most demanding of the three sports that make up triathlon. If you fall into any of the above categories, or perhaps another one that just says, "swim, no," then duathlon is for you. And hopefully, this book will be for you too.

For this book is the first one of the twenty-first century to be devoted entirely to duathlon training and racing. And it comes out at a time when the national multisport racing governing body, USA Triathlon (USAT) is undertaking a program to further develop and promote duathlon at all levels. As it happens, that program is described in chapter 2 of this book. There are many folks like myself who do both duathlons and triathlons. There are many folks who get started in multisport racing by doing duathlons first. And there are many others who do duathlons exclusively. But whatever category you see yourself in, this book can help you. For its focus is on duathlon exclusively, as a sport that stands on its own, right next to triathlon. It is designed to work for you if you are just starting out and also if you have been in the sport for some time but feel that you need to develop a more organized, focused approach to what you are doing.

In chapter 1, I introduce you to the sport and its several variants. Chapter 2 is from USAT, providing a brief review of the history of the duathlon and a look ahead at what USAT is doing to bring it up to the level it deserves. Chapter 3 introduces you to the element of training and preparation that for me always comes first: "Focusing Your Mind," the mental work that must be done if you are going to be successful in the physical part. Chapter 4 shows you how to find and choose your races intelligently, whether you are just starting out or have been at it for a while. Chapter 5 helps you to get ready to train, while chapter 6 shows you how to do that without being overwhelmed. You should know right now that you can safely do what is called a sprint-distance duathlon (a 2- to 3-mile run, 12- to 18-mile bike, 2- to 3-mile run), finishing happily and healthily, on as little as three-and-a-half hours of training altogether, just as long as you don't try to go too fast in the race.

Chapter 7 covers technique while chapter 8 does the same for equipment. Chapter 9 is devoted entirely to the "Day at the Races." Chapter 10 shows you how to make duathlon a central part of living a healthy lifestyle, while chapter 11 concludes the book with a consideration of special experiences that I have had doing duathlons, both short and long, and from myself and others, some philosophy and some humor. I hope that you will enjoy it and that it will help get you on the road to being able to finish happily and healthily, whether it's your first race or your fiftieth.

One does not do books like these without lots of help and inspiration. First, many thanks to my editor at Lyons Press/Globe Pequot Press, Keith Wallman, first for having the vision to see the future for this book, and then for a superb, what I like to call "old-timey" editing job. I also want to thank my copy editor for this book, Carol Kopec, who did such an outstanding job for me, as well as Kirsten Livingston, layout artist; Sheryl Kober, designer; Ellen Urban, project editor; and Sara Baker, digital/social media marketing manager. To my agent, Rita Rosenkrantz, I extend my gratidude for her top-drawer representation, past, present, and future. I want to thank the leadership of USA Triathlon, my new friend Rob Urbach, CEO, and my longtime friend Tim Yount, COO, for their encouragement along the way and of course for the contribution of chapter 2. Thanks too to my close friends and supporters over the years at USAT, both on the race courses and off them, Fred Dyrek and Amanda Duke, who run our national events program, and Jayme Ramson, our magazine and online media manager.

I thank also my friend Dan Honig, president of the New York Triathlon Club, stalwart of multisport racing almost since its inception, and one of the major early developers of duathlon (way back then called "biathlon") for his friendship and support since my early days as a tri- and duathlete, and for graciously authoring the foreword for this book. Then there are my thanks to all of those triathletes and duathletes who over the years have approached me at and even during the races, and have written to me, to let me know personally that my writings have helped them. It always gives me a thrill to have someone tell me directly that my work has affected their lives in a positive way.

Finally, I acknowledge the permission to use selections from previous writings of mine from Healthy Learning/ Coaches Choice publishers; Lippincott, Williams and Williams; *USA Triathlon Magazine* (Jayme Ramson, magazine and online media manager); and the *American Medical Athletics Association Journal* (Barbara Baldwin, dear friend and managing editor, who manages to keep me afloat in my position as editor-in-chief of the journal).

CHAPTER 1

What Is Duathlon?

Duathlon is a form of multisport distance racing—doing two or more sports in the same race—that gained traction not too long after the first popular form, triathlon, was developed in the mid-1970s. Triathlon, the swim-bike-run race, is by far the most common variant of multisport racing. Duathlon, originally known by a variety of names, came to some prominence in the 1980s, but in the 1990s fell to a distinct second-class status compared with triathlon. However, in the second decade of the 2000s, duathlon is making a strong comeback, in major part because of an organized push by our multisport racing national governing body, USA Triathlon. In chapter 2 of this book, you will find a full description of the USAT program for bringing duathlon racing back to national prominence.

In contrast to triathlon, duathlon involves only two sports, with either two or three race segments. In the three-segment duathlon, one of the two sports is done twice. The most common form of duathlon is a three-segment event, run-bike-run. In *Duathlon Training and Racing for Ordinary Mortals®*, we will devote most of our attention to that form. There are other variants, like aquathlon, a three-segment run-swim-run race, and AquaVelo (or aqua-bike), a two-segment swim-bike race. But most duathlons do not involve swimming. That is one of the primary reasons why the form was originally developed back in the mid-1980s. For the nonswimmers, it provided a very nice alternative to triathlon. And for triathletes in the colder climes, it provided for a longer multisport racing season.

The most common distances for the duathlon are 2 to 3 miles for each of the two run segments and 12 to 18 miles on the bike. This formula is more or less equivalent to the sprint triathlons that are becoming ever more popular (a quarter- to half-mile swim, a 12- to 18-mile bike and a 2- to 3-mile run). What we'll thus call the sprint-distance duathlons are widely held around the United States, either as freestanding races or in conjunction with a triathlon at a large racing event.

While for some people the duathlon serves as an entryway to triathlon racing, there are certainly many multisport athletes who stay just with duathlon. Then there are many others, like myself, who do both types of races in the course of the same season. The duathlon format also appeals to race directors since, compared to triathlons, they are easier and cheaper to set up, manage, and insure. The number of competitors in a duathlon usually ranges between fifty and four hundred, although there are occasionally larger races as well. On present duathlon courses, especially if the first run were to be started in waves—as is the swim in the larger triathlons—a significant increase in numbers could be accommodated.

There are run-bike-run duathlons longer than the sprint version, too. USA Triathlon hosts a national short-course and long-course championship each year, races that qualify athletes to attend their respective International Triathlon Union (ITU) Duathlon World Championships. (The ITU is the international governing body for multisport distance racing.) The 2011 USAT Duathlon National Championship race consisted of two 5-kilometer runs surrounding a 35-kilometer bike. For 2012, USAT added a sprint-distance duathlon to its age-group nationals: 2.5-kilometer run, 17-kilometer bike, and 2.5-kilometer run. Meanwhile, the ITU Duathlon World's short-course event consists of a 10-kilometer run, a 40-kilometer bike, and a 5-kilometer run. (It is somewhat similar to the short course, or Olympic-distance triathlon: a 1.5-kilometer swim, a 40-kilometer bike, and a 10-kilometer run.) The ITU short course duathlon worlds have a sprint-distance event as well.

Reflecting the increasing popularity of duathlon from 2005 to 2010, the 2010 Duathlon Age-Group Nationals, held in Richmond, Virginia, (in which I participated) was sold out, with about 1,800 competitors. For the 2011 race, held in Tucson—harder to get to for the sport's many eastern competitors—entries fell to about six hundred, but around a thousand are expected for the 2012 duathlon nationals in the same location.

Moving up the distance ladder, there is the 15-kilometer run, 60-kilometer bike, and 7.5-kilometer run of the worldwide Powerman Duathlon Series events. At the pinnacle is the Powerman Zofingen, held in Switzerland each year. This race, due to its grueling nature in the Swiss Alps, is often compared to an ironman triathlon (2.4-mile swim, 112-mile bike, and 26.2-mile marathon run), and attracts hundreds of athletes and thousands of spectators from around the world. The race consists of a 10-kilometer run, 150-kilometer bike, and 30-kilometer run.

Other Two-sport Races

As mentioned, there are several other two-sport distance races, although they are much less common than the run-bike-run duathlon. The aquathlon is a run-swim-run event, most often held over relatively short distances. For example, the USA Triathlon National and the International Triathlon Union World Championship Aquathlons consist of a 2.5-kilometer run, a 1-kilometer swim, and another 2.5-kilometer run. Then there is the aquabike or AquaVelo, a two-leg swim-bike event. Originally, beginning in the early 2000s, aquabikes were held exclusively in combination with half-ironman triathlons (the distances being a 1.2-mile swim followed by a 56-mile bike). But moving into the second decade of the twenty-first century, aquabike races at shorter distances are becoming more popular. One can also occasionally find local swim-run and run-bike races at short distances. However, the dominant form of two-sport racing is the sprint-distance run-bike-run duathlon, of which I have done more than eighty, as well as a few longer ones (in three cases much longer ones). The duathlon is the multisport race for the many non-swimmers among us. Thus, the bulk of this book will focus on "doin' the du."

Is the Run-Bike-Run Duathlon for You?

Is the du' right for you? The answer is yes, if you want to get into multisport racing, but:

1. You are an unskilled or nonswimmer or simply not thrilled with the idea of swimming, and/or,

2. You don't look forward to training in three sports (two are plenty for you), and/or,

3. You are looking for a shorter multisport event that is not as demanding as a sprint triathlon (because of the swimming) but still presents a good challenge for you, and/or,

4. You are interested in a multisport event that is logistically simpler to undertake than a triathlon and/or,

5. You are most comfortable on the bike and are perfectly happy to do the bulk of your training on it.

If so, you are the ideal candidate for Doin' the Du.

Indeed, the sprint-distance run-bike-run duathlon is a fun race that is quite manageable for all of us ordinary mortals. The logistics are much simpler than they are for triathlon. Along with no swim, there is no swim stuff to be concerned with. Then, think about the transitions between one segment and the next, which are an essential part of multisport racing. For duathlon you need to learn only how to do the run-bike and bike-run transitions. Furthermore, because in the nonswimming du's there is no worry about water temperature, in many parts of the country the duathlon season is considerably longer than the triathlon season.

Duathlon is a distance-racing sport for every kind of competitor. There are duathletes who go fast, and more power to them. But for me, one of the best things about duathlon (and triathlon, too) is that it's for everyone—fast, slow, and in between. Before I became a triathlete and a duathlete too, I had been a small cruising boat sailor. I did club racing on occasion. If you didn't finish among the top three boats, that was it. Getting around the course successfully didn't count for anything. But in multisport racing, getting around the course successfully is a great objective and it *does* count. You did it! You got there! Even if you finished last, you finished ahead of everyone you know who didn't get out on the course. Since I was slow when I started out in multisport racing, I made my first objective simply to finish, as I like to say, "happily and healthily."

Now, as I have gotten older, there are fewer and fewer men in my age group still racing, especially on my home turf in the New York City metropolitan area, where the age group began to thin out fairly early. And so, beginning in my early sixties, I began coming home with plaques for first-to-third place age-group finishes. For the most part, that simply required getting to the starting line and crossing the finish line (and still does). Plaques are fun, I have to admit it. But my primary objective in each and every race is still, twenty-nine years after I started, to finish the race happily and healthily, regardless of where I place either overall or in my age group.

To race happily and healthily, you might ask yourself: How much do I need to train? We will get into training in detail starting with chapter 5, but if you are in basic aerobic shape—doing two to three hours per week in an aerobic sport like running or cycling—you can be ready for your first sprint-distance duathlon with a thirteen-week program in which you average a total of three and a half hours per week. If you are starting from scratch, not working out at all right now or working out irregularly, you'll need just thirteen weeks—maximum—to get yourself ready to start the sprint-distance duathlon training program mentioned above. We will go over this "starting from scratch," foundation program, in detail in chapter 6.

My message here is that you don't need to quit your job or abandon your family to join in this sport. However, you do have to have your goals clearly in mind, and those goals have to be reasonable and realistic for you (see chapter 3). And then you have to be regular and consistent in your training (see chapter 5). That is, you have to be focused. If you are, you can do it and have a great time at the same time!

Some History: A Personal Perspective[*]

Multisport distance racing has become increasingly popular around the world during the past thirty-plus years. At the International Triathlon Union (ITU) Duathlon World Championships, held in a different country each year, more than thirty nations are represented by national teams. In the United States, membership in USA-Triathlon grew from a few thousand in the late 1980s to more than 150,000 at the beginning of the 2011 season. (My own membership number, which goes back to USAT's predecessor organization, the Triathlon Federation-USA, which I joined in the mid-1980s, is 3271. I am very proud of that fact.)

While the essence of multisport racing for the amateur has changed little, if at all, there have been some important developments over the past decades. The total number of multisport races, at a wide range of distances, has increased markedly. Second, the recent resurgence of duathlons, as

---

* See also chapter 2.

well as the widespread popularity of "sprint" triathlons (one-quarter- to one-half-mile swim, 10- to 15-mile bike, 3- to 5-mile run), has made it much easier for first-timers to get into multisport racing and for recreational, relatively light training multi-sport athletes like me to stay in it.

The two-sport variant of triathlon first appeared in the mid-1980s, under a variety of names: byathlon, run-bike-run, cyruthon (cycle-run), and the name that stuck for a while: biathlon. In the early days, the most common format was run-bike, but there were also run-bike-run and bike-run variants. The sport quickly evolved, however, to focus exclusively on the run-bike-run format. The biathlon was originally viewed by one of its principal developers, my good friend Daniel Honig, president of the New York Triathlon Club (NYTC, originally named the Big Apple Triathlon Club, BATC), as a way to extend the multisport racing season in both the spring and the fall.

As noted, it quickly was seen as an entryway into multisport racing for weak or nonswimmers, some of whom might then stay with the form indefinitely. Dan had originally organized the BATC back in 1983, running triathlons for a four-month summer season. By 1984 he had added run-bike-run biathlons to his race schedule. His initial idea was to extend the multisport racing season in the New York Metropolitan area. He quickly saw that for a number of athletes he had developed an alternative multisport race. Despite the ups and downs of the sport nationally (see chapter 2), thanks to Dan Honig's continuous efforts, the biathlon/duathlon has maintained a prominent place on the New York metropolitan area's race calendar. Every year there are three races in Central Park, three to four in the outer boroughs of New York City, and several more at nearby locations in the region. "When I was a boy" in multisport terms, I did my first biathlon (my third multi-sport race overall) in May 1984 at the old Floyd Bennett Field (a former Naval air station) in Brooklyn, New York (in the rain, as I recall).

I also happen to have competed in what was the first Triathlon Federation USA official Biathlon National Championship, held in New York City's Central Park in November, 1986. (In those days all those races had open entries.) A second one was held in November 1987. Big names, like Mark Allen and Kenny Souza, came in for those races. To this day I do two to four of Dan's duathlons each season.

Dan, quite the iconoclast, continued to call the event the "biathlon" into 2011, when he did formally change the name of his races to "duathlon." Internationally, the name change to "duathlon" came about in the mid-1990s, when the International Triathlon Union applied for the inclusion of triathlon in the Olympic Games. As the campaign got under way, even though there was no idea of including the run-bike biathlon in the Olympics as well, the need to come up with a new name for triathlon's two-sport offspring became apparent. In the Winter Olympics, there is a well-established Nordic event that combines cross-country skiing and target shooting, also known as the "biathlon." Understandably, the International Biathlon Union did not want even the possibility that there might be another event in the Olympics, summer or winter, sharing their event's name. So, using a Latin rather than a Greek prefix while maintaining the Greek root, the name "duathlon" for the run-bike (and eventually other two-sport events) races was created.

There are no firm historical data on numbers of duathlon participants in the United States. However, it is widely felt that, outside of the New York metropolitan region and a few others, beginning in the first half of the 1990s, duathlon went into a decline in both number of races and total participants. As USAT said on its website (www.usatriathlon.org/disciplines/duathlon) in July of 2010:

The sport of duathlon in the United States hit an all-time high in the 1980s when big-time sponsors such as Coors Lite produced [duathlon] series that had thousands participating in a single race. Though duathlon slipped in numbers when corporate sponsorship faded [in the early '90s], the sport enjoyed resurgence in the late '90s and early 2000s with the Dannon Duathlon series and duathlon races growing across the country.

Unfortunately for athletes and race directors alike, the Dannon Duathlon series bowed out in 2004. [Nevertheless, for reasons that are not entirely clear] even with the fall of the corporate sponsorships, the US has witnessed a growth in sanctioned duathlons in 2007 and 2008. . . . Participants can find events ranging from local, low key races to big time production events. . . . USA-T is committed to increasing the number of participants in duathlon events and is working with race directors to ensure events are spread out throughout the season [emphasis added].

This commitment to the duathlon occurs within the context of very significant growth in multisport racing overall at the time (USA Triathlon Life, Summer 2010). As noted in that article, the Sporting Goods Manufacturers Association (SGMA) estimated that in 2010 there were about two million unique individuals entered in on-road triathlons and more than 900,000 unique individuals entered in off-road triathlons. According to SGMA, these numbers reflect over 148 percent and over 92 percent growth rates respectively for on-road and off-road triathlons since 2007. According to former USA-Triathlon CEO Skip Gilbert, "The continued growth of the multisport lifestyle across all disciplines and distances is a strong reflection of this country's desire to focus on healthy living. Incorporating not one but a multitude of sports into an individual's training and competition schedule has simply exploded in popularity, and we at USA-Triathlon are proud to be able to support these individuals' passions."

As of 2011, USA Triathlon began a major effort to promote duathlon racing. Along with the history of the sport from the USAT perspective, the organization's efforts are presented in the next chapter.

CHAPTER 2

USA Triathlon and Duathlon*

In the early 1980s the United States began to see astonishing development in multisport racing. It had begun on a small scale in San Diego in the mid-1970s with the appearance of the multisport race that quickly came to be known as triathlon—swimming, cycling, and running. Duathlon (then known by several other names) made its appearance shortly thereafter. The popularity of duathlon and triathlon events on the West Coast drove demand for multisport races in other parts of the country. Sports enthusiasts traveled vast distances to participate in what is known today as the multisport movement.

Due to the rapid growth in both triathlon and duathlon racing, many athletes and race directors expressed a need for leadership, direction, and development that could come only from a national governing body. To meet that expressed need, in February 1982 James Gayton and John Disterdick founded the US Triathlon Association. In March 1982, Jarold Johnson, Michael Gilmore, and Penny Little followed by forming the American Triathlon Association. A month later, the two organizations met and merged as the US Triathlon Association. Beginning in 1983, the association focused much of its effort on national-event production and race sanctioning, including

* The original text for chapter 2 was written by Wendy Peel, sport development coordinator, and Tim Yount, chief operating officer, USA Triathlon, and is used with permission.

the provision of race liability insurance at reasonable rates. The organization established insurance coverage and supported multisport race directors, which in turn supported the growth of the multisport movement. In that first year, 1983, there were about one thousand sanctioned multisport events.

By August 1983, the original organizers had changed the name of the governing body to the Triathlon Federation USA, to be known colloquially as Tri-Fed. In 1985, the Triathlon Federation USA established a board of directors to govern itself and the development of the multisport movement. Tri-Fed collected dues from members and sanctioning fees from the race directors, and thus was able to hire a professional staff. Over the next five years, board and staff working together developed and implemented a program to support the growing sport and the development of the national governing body. The key goals were increasing the number and quality of sanctioned events, membership growth, improved customer service for both athletes and race directors, improved educational programs and resources, offering sponsored national championship events, and continuing sport development efforts. As these program initiatives were unveiled, the need for a program to support high-performance athletes came to be a critical priority for the organization.

In 1990, the Triathlon Federation USA submitted a comprehensive application for membership to the United States Olympic Committee (USOC). Then, in 1991, the International Olympic Committee (IOC) recognized the International Triathlon Union (ITU) as the sole transnational governing body for the sport. Three years later, the IOC decided to add triathlon as an Olympic sport, beginning with the 2000 Summer Games held in Sydney, Australia. The Triathlon Federation USA changed its name in 1996 to USA Triathlon, thus making it consistent with those of the other national governing bodies that are USOC members, such as USA Track and Field, and USA Swimming.

As of 2011, USA Triathlon proudly served as the national governing body for the sports of triathlon, duathlon, aquathlon, aquabike, winter triathlon, and paratriathlon in the United States. USA Triathlon sanctioned more than 3,500 races and connected with 150,000-plus members each year, making it the largest multisport organization in the world. In addition to its work with athletes, coaches, and race directors on the grassroots level, USA Triathlon provides leadership and support to elite athletes competing at international events, including the ITU World Championships, the Pan American Games, and, of course, the Summer Olympic Games. USA Triathlon is a proud member of the International Triathlon Union and the United States Olympic Committee.

Historical Developments in Duathlon: A USAT Perspective

Duathlon participation was one of the driving forces for the creation of Tri-Fed early in the development of the multisport movement. Strong athlete numbers allowed event production companies to build relationships with national-level partners who, in return, supported the events' robust budgets and strong marketing campaigns. In the late 1980s and early 1990s, the Coors Brewing Company supported a multiple-race duathlon series, the Coors Light Series. It was common for the series to draw six hundred to seven hundred athletes in a single race, as many of their events were located in larger markets that ensured large athlete draws. Many top professionals sharpened their multisport teeth with this series. However, duathlon participation slipped in numbers when the Coors Light Series corporate sponsorship ended in 1994.

Duathlon then enjoyed resurgence in the late 1990s and early 2000s with the appearance of the Dannon Duathlon Series. The Dannon events were located in markets where grocery-store support was greatest. Unfortunately, the Dannon Duathlon Series ended in 2004. However, even with the absence of a national duathlon series, the United States still witnessed growth in the number of sanctioned duathlon events. In 2008, USA Triathlon sanctioned 400 duathlons in forty-eight states, followed by 441 in 2009, and 475 in 2010. With the growth in the number of sanctioned events, athletes were able to find duathlon races ranging from local, low-key events to large scale production competitions. Participants who wished to compete on the regional and national level could do so through a set of USAT Duathlon Regional Championships and the USAT Duathlon National Championship, both held annually.

The USAT Duathlon Short Distance National Championship has been in existence since 1989. Participant numbers for this event have ranged from 285 to 1,805 athletes. When USAT added a Long Distance Duathlon National Championship in 1996, numbers varied between 200 and 1,300 competitors. In Richmond, Virginia, in 2009, USAT supported an all-in-one-venue national championship comprising an off-road duathlon, a youth competition, and the popular standard-distance event. Total participation soared to 1,700 athletes. That number was eclipsed in 2010 when 1,805 athletes competed in the Duathlon National Championship in the same location. With a shift to Tucson, Arizona, there was a dip in attendance to 580 athletes. This precipitous drop in participation, probably related to the Southwestern location and the state of the US economy, is typical for a sport such as duathlon; it takes time for new national-championship venues to spawn interest and invigorate the discipline in a new region. The present plan foresees participation numbers in 2013 that will rival those of Richmond in 2009 and 2010.

In the early 1990s, USA Triathlon and its ten regional councils had recognized the growth in the sport and developed a Duathlon Regional Championship in each of the regions. This development benefited duathletes who desired to test themselves against those who resided in their competition area. In 2011, seven of the ten USAT designated regions hosted a Duathlon Regional Championship.

A critical component of duathlon's development over time has been creating opportunity for amateurs to qualify for the ITU Duathlon World Championships—gaining membership in what is called Team USA for the sport. Since 1990, nearly ten thousand athletes have competed at these international events. More recently, athletes have qualified through the Duathlon National Championships for a chance to compete for Team USA and represent their country at the ITU Duathlon World Championships at three different events, held at two different venues: the short- and standard-distance races held at one and the long-course duathlon held separately (check the ITU website, www.triathlon.org/events; search on "duathlon" for details).

As the number of sanctioned events grew at the local, regional, national, and international level, the need for formal athlete recognition grew also. Thus, a national individual rankings program was developed, based on weighted race performance. At first, all multisport athletes were ranked together, but by the mid-1990s, duathlon rankings were separated from those of triathlon. Duathletes were then able to compare their rankings with those of duathletes from around the country. Another program that benefited the growth of the sport was the crowning of Duathletes of the Year. Male and female Duathletes of the Year have been named since 1999 in the overall, junior, masters, and grand masters categories. These two programs have helped increase participation numbers for the sport of duathlon.

The latest development in the sport has been an expanded branding effort. Since 2005, duathlon apparel has been offered through a USAT merchandiser. The apparel has been sold online, at nationals, and at United States-based world championship events. Event directors have also created duathlon branding around their own events. This branding opportunity has supported necessary differentiation between the sister sports of triathlon and duathlon.

The Master Duathlon Plan and the Future of Duathlon

Dedicated to the development of new program ideas and because duathletes comprise the second-largest constituency group among USA Triathlon's membership, the USAT board of directors appointed a Duathlon Committee in late 2000. Consisting of duathletes, coaches, and race directors, the committee made many decisions regarding national championship events and Team USA from 2005 to 2008. Focus then shifted to grassroots development in the United States at the local level. In October 2008, USAT staff proposed a redefinition of the mission of the Duathlon Committee: to develop a comprehensive program to promote the growth of the sport at the community/local level. The group began work in 2009 and by 2011 had produced a master duathlon plan to organically support the growth of the sport and to achieve the long-term potential of duathlon as a major actor on the national multisport stage. In its plan, the committee identified both short- and long-term goals and objectives for the period spanning the second decade of the twenty-first century.

At the 2011 USAT Duathlon National Championships in Tucson, Arizona, Tonya Armstrong, who co-chaired the committee along with Faye Yates, presented the master duathlon plan to an assembly of athletes, coaches, race directors, and several members of the USAT Board of Directors. In her presentation, Armstrong identified the short-term goals for the 2011 and 2012 seasons to an eager and attentive crowd of duathlon enthusiasts. The first point of emphasis was the development of a regional series built around the duathlon sectional championships as designated by the regional councils. A series composed of the top sectionally identified duathlons would support not only the standard short-distance duathlon ("sprint-distance" in the rest of this book) but even shorter distances that multisport novices could master. The consensus was that a shorter distance event would attract new interest and drive participation.

The second short-term goal of the plan was to increase promotional activities through expanded relationships with duathlon/triathlon clubs and other local organizations, along with website and media outlets, using the USAT national office and the ten USAT regions. Four objectives were designed to promote the sport at the grassroots level: First, the committee and USAT staff would continue to build relationships with multisport clubs nationwide and implement duathlon training and racing programs at the community level. Second, the committee would work closely with the USAT National Office to set up a specific website address that would direct athletes to the duathlon section of the USAT website, as well as to other areas of the USA Triathlon site where entry-level information for duathlon would be located.

Third, the committee/staff team would investigate the availability of and then purchase booth space at large running and cycling expositions across the country to promote local, regional, and national duathlon races. The booth presentations would be supported by video from current USAT Duathlon national competitions, event brochures and calendars, as well as USA Triathlon promotional items that have the potential to make duathlon attractive to its largest potential new markets: athletes who are already both road and off-road running and cycling racers. The final short-term objective was to build a community duathlon training program for both youth and adults that could be administered by local YMCAs, YWCAs, Boys & Girls Clubs of America, PALs, fitness centers and health clubs, as well as neighborhood recreation centers. The committee also established additional long-term goals that would be further developed in the following three to five years. The first goal was to develop and implement a youth duathlon program. The staff would work directly with the regional councils to form relationships with multisport clubs, coaches, and race directors to develop a comprehensive youth program that could be emulated by any community in the United States. To support the programs, USAT would encourage its race director constituency to organize local youth duathlon events across the nation. This program would ensure growth through the developmental pipeline.

Over the long term, the committee also hoped to create a collegiate duathlon plan. The group would work closely with USAT staff as well as the USAT Collegiate Committee to build a robust program and encourage the growth of the sport at the collegiate level. The program would attempt to emulate the success of the USAT's already existing Collegiate Triathlon Program.

A final element of the master duathlon plan was to encourage USA Triathlon race directors to host duathlons simultaneously with triathlons. Such pairings were already being done by a number of race directors around the country. The swim leg of the standard Olympic-distance triathlon, the most popular variant of that sport, is 1.5 kilometers. Many duathlons include a 5-kilometer first run leg. The times are amazingly consistent for both, at every level of the competition spectrum. By having the first two segments of each competition occur at the same time, race directors can have all athletes compete over the same bike-and-run distances for the final two disciplines of the event. Not only does this keep athletes in the heat of several unexpected battles on the playing field, but it simplifies the time line that many directors face as part of the local permitting process.

In 2011, the Duathlon Committee concluded that the list of goals above comprises the key elements necessary if duathlon participation across the country is to grow significantly.

The duathlon committee and USAT staff firmly believe that through this cooperative effort they have developed a plan that will produce growth in the sport that will take it to a level of participation well beyond that seen in its three-decades-long history so far.

How You Can Help the Sport to Grow

Are you already passionate about duathlon? If you are a beginner, are you already thinking that you might become a passionate duathlete? USA Triathlon and the Duathlon Committee are looking for volunteers to support the key initiatives from the Master Duathlon Plan. In the last thirty years, USA Triathlon has been fortunate to have committed athletes, coaches, and race directors who are willing to help organically grow the sport and ensure the long-term potential of duathlon. Individuals who are enthusiastic about duathlon and who would like to volunteer are encouraged to contact USA Triathlon directly at membership@usatriathlon.org or visit the website at www.usatriathlon.org.

CHAPTER 3

It All Starts with Your Mind

One of my dear friends is a man named Bob Roses. I taught skiing with Bob for about ten years at the Breckenridge (Colorado) Ski and Ride School beginning in 1996. Bob, an experienced ski instructor, was fond of saying, "Skiing is 90 percent mental—and the rest is in your head."

"What do you mean?" you might ask. "Isn't skiing all about technique?"

"Well, yes," Bob would say, "of course it's about technique. But you will never be able to get to the technique, much less master it, unless and until you've got your mind wrapped around the subject."

It is absolutely the same thing for Doin' the Du.

Mark Allen, who won the Hawaii Ironman six times through 1993, once described winning that race as a "mental exercise in pain management." As someone who has finished an ironman-distance triathlon (2.4-mile swim, 112 on the bike, then a marathon) three times, I can tell you that Mark has that one right. However, let me assure you that for recreational duathletes, doing sprint-distance races only very occasionally becomes a "pain management" issue, and usually only if you are trying to go too fast. But for any duathlete in any duathlon, and more importantly in preparing for it, the mental work is at least as significant as the physical work. You won't be able to do the latter effectively unless you have first done the former. The key element in making sure that you are appropriately trained is mental discipline. Then, the longer your race, the more important your mind power becomes in relation to your body power.

Except for those folks at the front of the pack, who are technical bike riders or fast runners, there is little physical or athletic skill involved in doing the primary duathlon sports: cycling and running. Left, right, left, right is the name of the game for running until you get to the point where you can, and want to, go fast. Just about any of us can ride a bike, and although technique becomes important again when you want to go fast, and when you are going up and down hills, around tight turns, and pedaling in bike traffic, it is not *athletic* skill that is involved. We're not talking about the team sports, or tennis or golf here. And while we all perspire profusely on a hot day, it is not the perspiration per se which gets us through the race. It's our mind—our mental determination to get properly trained, and our determination to meet the race-day challenge—that sees us through to the end. For the successful duathlete, mind training is at least as important as body training.

Starting Out, If You Haven't Done Anything Like This Before

Some of you will take the path to duathlon through one of its two sports. Maybe you are already road racing on foot or on the bike, and you want to try something new. Others of you are regular exercisers, and perhaps you've decided to spice up your training programs with a race. Maybe you think that doing one involving two sports, not just one, would be a fun way to do it. Still others of you are in a third group of readers; you're not regularly exercising now, but for one reason or another have decided that you would like to do a Du' and know, or should know, that you will have to become regular exercisers first if you are going to be successful in your new endeavor. Let me address this last group first with the hope that members of the first two will find some benefit from the discussion as well.

You cannot become a duathlete without first becoming a regular exerciser, as you will realize when you get to the training chapter. Becoming a regular exerciser is a challenge. But have faith. There are millions of people who have met the challenge. You can too. The first thing to recognize is the following: *The hard part of regular exercise is the regular, not the exercise.* Of almost all the personal health-promoting behaviors that you can undertake, like becoming a nonsmoker or learning to eat in a healthy way, regular exercise is one of only two endeavors that takes extra time for as long as you are doing it. (The other one that comes to mind is becoming a recovering alcoholic and going to group/meetings on an ongoing basis to stay sober.)

The second thing to recognize is that if all it took to become a regular exerciser were information on *why* exercise is "good for you," and *what to do* in terms of sports and workout schedules, then just about everyone would do it. The media bombards us with both kinds of that information all day, every day, and yet the bulk of our population is getting ever heavier and ever more sedentary. So just knowing that exercise is "good for you" and knowing "what to do" is hardly good enough to get you or anyone else going. This is where your mind comes in.

My starting point as a regular exerciser began with an experience that I had at the Cobo Conference Center in Detroit, Michigan, back in October 1980. At 8:30 one morning, I was walking up a one-flight ramp to get to a meeting room where I would give a presentation on lobbying government officials. I was huffing and puffing by the time I got to the top of the ramp, an experience that, as a nonathlete at the age of forty-three, I was having with increasing frequency. "OK," I said to myself. "The time has come. I've got to get in shape. I'm going to start running. I know I'm going to hate it, but I've got to do it, three times a week." And so I did.

Why that time, when I was huffing and puffing? Why not a year or two before, or a year or two afterward? Who knows, but it did happen, at that time.

I was off and running, starting out with Jim Fixx's program from his great book, *The Complete Runner*. I soon found that what I had thought might be a chore, actually was becoming enjoyable. Then a love for racing developed when, beginning in the spring of 1982, I started road racing. That season I gradually worked my way up the ladder from the 5 kilometer to the 10k distance. It was in the spring of 1983 that I set my sights on becoming a triathlete, training all summer to get ready. On September 17, 1983, at Sag Harbor, New York, I did the second running of the Mighty Hamptons Triathlon. I did my first duathlon (then called "biathlon," as you already know), my third multisport race overall, in the rain at the old Floyd Bennett Field in Brooklyn, New York, in May 1984. "You were willing to suffer through a race in the rain in only your third one?" you might ask. Oh yes. I was hooked after my first one. There it is again, the mental part. Getting "hooked"—and, yes, there are many positive addictions—can be as much a mental process as a physical one. For you, getting going may not be the result of any specific experience, but rather for reasons that you could not put a finger on, you have thought, or will think: "You know, I would really like to try exercising regularly. I've got friends who do it and, boy, it seems to produce really good outcomes for them."

Now, the way *not* to get started is as follows. There are many people, and perhaps you are one of them, who have not exercised for some time or perhaps ever. You woke up one morning, put on an old pair of sneakers that were lurking in the back of the closet, and went out for a quick 4-mile run. Or you went to the gym and started lifting some weights (the heavier the better, no?) or sat down on the rowing machine (pulling faster is better, no?) for half an hour.

Oh, the pain the next morning! Oh, the stiffness as you try to walk a flight of stairs. It's enough to make a person stop.

But let's try again. This time, let's first *think* about what we're going to do and why. Let's spend the time it takes to *mobilize our motivation*, a mental process, before we start engaging in the physical one. Let's plan what we're going to do and then adopt the right kind of program to help us get there.

That's right, to achieve success—even as a regular exerciser—you need to do some mental work before you ever lace up your running shoes or hop on that dusty bike in your garage or storeroom. So let's get started, not with any physical exercise right away, but with some mental exercise.

The Basic Eight of Regular Exercise

As you surely know by now, the successful duathlete at any level trains/exercises regularly. Over the thirty-plus years that I have been a regular exerciser and a writer about the subject, I have put together a Basic Eight of Regular Exercise. These tenets have helped me to keep on truckin'. Given some thought, they will hopefully help you, too. Several of them are important enough that I repeat them once or twice in other parts of the book.

1. There are many reasons for exercising regularly. Most folks who do it will tell you that the most important ones are that regular exercise makes you feel better and feel better about yourself, makes you look better and look better to yourself, as well as to others. Those are certainly my principal reasons, even though as a preventive medicine doctor, I know that there are plenty of health-promoting reasons to do it, too.

2. Indeed, regular exercise can reduce your risk of heart disease, obesity, high blood pressure, stroke, certain kinds of cancer, diabetes, osteoporosis, and even depression and chronic anxiety. There are no guarantees here, but the *risk* goes down for getting all of these. Regular exercise is also very helpful in treating and managing many of the same conditions.

3. The *best exercise* for you is the exercise that is best for *you*. There are numerous choices. One size does not fit all. This applies to duathlon racing as well as to training for it.

4. The hard part of regular exercise is the regular, not the exercise.

5. It is *gradual* change that leads to *permanent* change.

6. Explore your limits; recognize your limitations.

7. Effective mobilization of your motivation is the key to long-term success, first as a regular exerciser and then as a duathlete.

8. We can never be perfect; we can always get better.

Training the Mind for Duathlon

The importance and the power of the mind in duathlon is nowhere more evident than in training. Most training sessions should either be fun in themselves or at least acceptable, if for no other reason than that you know in order to race you have to train, and you *do* want to race. But you need to train, day after most days, week after week, and stick to that schedule.

You need to be able to go out for a scheduled workout in the morning, not just when you're full of vim and vigor, but also when you awaken feeling very sleepy. (For me, exercise time is in the morning; for you it may be at another time of the day. You have to pick what is going to work best for you.) Even at only four to five hours of training per week (which is what the Doin' the Du Training Program for the sprint-distance duathlon requires), there are still times that you've got to get out there but you really don't want to. That requires the mental discipline that we'll discuss below. You'll also need mental discipline not to *over*train. Knowing when enough is enough to achieve the results that you want is essential. When it comes to potential long-term damage to your body and also your racing career, overdoing it at times can be more harmful than under-doing it. And even when your training and your racing season are going well, you need the mental discipline to say, from time to time, "let's take it easy this week, or let's even take the week off. I know that my conditioning won't disappear overnight [and it won't], and my muscles surely could use some rest."

Mobilizing Your Motivation

What is the key to becoming a successful duathlete? It is the mental activity of *mobilizing your motivation* and keeping it mobilized, something that you will do multiple times: when you start out to become a regular exerciser, when you decide to do that first race, when (and if) you decide that you want to race on a regular basis, and when, once having decided that, you commit yourself to training regularly so that you can race regularly. If you are going to get to the stage where you are effectively using your mind in training, in racing, or even in stopping on a particular training day or during a particular race, you must first be motivated to become a regular exerciser, to start training to do that first race, and then perhaps go on to become a regular duathlete.

What Is Motivation?

In general terms, most people know what they are thinking about when they say "I've got to get motivated" or "my motivation is high for this one." But few of us can immediately put into words exactly what we mean when we use the term. Consider this definition:

Motivation is a state of mind characterized as: an emotion, feeling, desire, idea, or intellectual understanding, or a psychological, physiological, or health need mediated by a mental process, that leads to the taking of one or more actions.

Too long a definition for you? How about this one, which is the one that I happen to use on a regular basis when I am writing about or leading discussions on the subject:

Motivation is a mental process that connects a thought or a feeling with an action.

Thus, when we talk about either "being motivated" or "lacking motivation" to do something, like training for and participating in a duathlon, we are referring to the state of mind that will help us/push us to do it. As indicated by the linguistic relationship between the words "motivation" and "move," the former is always related to action. (Please note that we shall return to this subject in some more detail in chapter 10, in a discussion of how to apply this knowledge and understanding to leading a healthy lifestyle overall.)

The Ordinary Mortal's® Pathway to Mobilizing Motivation
To help you organize your approach to the process, I have developed what I call the Ordinary Mortal's® Pathway to Mobilizing

Motivation, or the OMPMM. This mental process has five stages. Whatever level of duathlon racing you have achieved, at any given time, you will find the OMPMM very helpful in keeping you going and keeping you focused. Once you learn the following five steps of the pathway, you will find yourself periodically taking them in a continuous feedback loop:

1. Assess yourself.

2. Define success for yourself.

3. Set goals.

4. Establish priorities.

5. Take control of the whole process.

We will discuss the OMPMM steps briefly here, and again in more detail in chapter 10. To make the process work best for you, I strongly suggest that, for each step in the pathway, you write down your thoughts.

1. Assess Yourself. If you want to get somewhere new, the first step is identifying and understanding your starting point. Self-assessment is asking yourself questions like, Where am I now? How did I get here? What would I like to change? What is going on in my life that would assist or deter me in becoming a regular exerciser and then a duathlete?

If you think about assessing yourself, you will notice that it is applicable to every stage of the exercising/racing adventure. If you are a beginning exerciser, it will help you define where you want to get first. If you are already a regular exerciser, thinking about becoming a duathlete, rationally and reasonably assessing yourself will help you to define what training program and what race or races you want to start out with. If you are an experienced racer, self-assessment at the end of each season, and sometimes in the middle of a season, is helpful in deciding what you want to do next, so that you will stay in the sport and keep on enjoying it—even if things aren't going so well at the time. And if your racing is going well, self-assessment to understand why is also very helpful.

2. Define Success. The second step on the Ordinary Mortal's® Pathway to Mobilizing Motivation is defining success for yourself. If the contemplated project is going to work for you, your definition of success has to be reasonable, it has to be rational, it has to be something that you can see yourself realistically achieving, given the amount of time you have available. What success means to you has to be answered in the context of you as a person, what your measure of your innate skills and capabilities is. Very importantly, you should avoid setting yourself up for failure. Defining success productively also includes giving yourself permission to fail, assuming that you really did try. As Dave Scott, one of the greatest triathletes of all time and a member of the USA Triathlon Hall of Fame, once said: "I encourage all . . . triathletes to reach for your goals, whether they be to win or just to try. The trying is everything."

3. Set Goals. Third along the OM Pathway is the central element of the whole process: goal setting. Your goals should be built upon your own definition of success for yourself: What is it that I want to do and why do I want to do it? If you ask yourself, *For whom do I want to do it?* the answer has to be *for yourself*, not for anyone else. "Other-motivation" simply does not work. That can easily lead to frustration, guilt, anger, then possibly injury, then quitting. You want none of these. Further, building upon your definition of what success is for *you*, what do you think you can *reasonably* and *rationally* expect to achieve as a goal or goals? (Note how the Three Rs—realistic, reasonable, and rational—keep reappearing in my thoughts on the subjects of motivation and goal setting.) And then, very importantly, to achieve your goals, what are the "give-ups" you have to make? What will you *not* be able to do with your time if you now devote some of it to racing and training for the races on a regular and consistent basis? Can you, do you want to, commit to those give-ups? Arriving at satisfactory answers to these questions is absolutely key. Doing so provides the focus and the concentration you must have in order to have the best chance of success in your chosen endeavor.

For duathlon racing specifically, what is it that you want to do in the sport and why do you want to do it? Again, what is it that you are reasonably capable of doing, given your athletic history and your reasonably achievable level of physical conditioning? Before you push a pedal or take a step, to become a successful duathlete on your own terms (whatever they may be), you need to have a clear vision of what you want to accomplish and why you want to accomplish it. All the while, you must be realistic, reasonable, and rational about your goals.

Do you want to simply finish, to go fast, to place in your age group, to win the race overall? Is finishing in the middle to the back of the pack acceptable? Is last okay, just as long as you finish, happily and healthily? (Hey, finishing last can be better than finishing sixth from last. I have done both, on more than one occasion! With the former, everyone knows who you are. With the latter you are completely anonymous!) Depending upon your equipment (primarily meaning your mind and body, not your bike), your commitment, and your available time, any of the above can be a reasonable goal. But to achieve any of them, in a sentence, you need to "have it clear in your mind just what it is you want to do, and just why you want to do it." That's goal setting.

Goals, of course, need not be related to specific races, to specific times, or to getting to the podium for an age-group award at the end of the race. Those are all important or can be. But unless you have an unusual set of skills and experience to begin with, they should probably be secondary to setting realistic and rational goals, like crossing the finish line happily and healthily, or just enjoying the whole experience, from setting up in the transition area to cheering at the awards ceremony, or finding out that yes, this is a place that I want to be on a somewhat regular basis. In fact, the subsequent achievement of race-specific goals depends precisely upon the *appropriate* setting of such realistic and rational *personal* goals first.

4. Establish Priorities. The fourth OMPMM step is to establish priorities among duathlon training and racing and your family, work, and social life. Too much of a good thing can be as damaging to your health and well-being as not enough. If you are not mentally and physically equipped to do it, and if you have too many other things going on in your life, too much racing can do as much harm as sitting on the couch. Establishing priorities among your specific goals, and then among those goals and the rest of your life is central to making the whole process work for you. If you have set multiple goals, what are their rankings? Which do you consider to be the most important to achieve? Which the least? If juggling of time among family, friends, other leisure time activities, and your job needs to be done, it will be very helpful to do some thinking about priority establishment.

5. Take Control. Finally, in order to mobilize your motivation, you must put yourself in charge of the whole process, adopt an "I can do this" attitude and perspective. Take control. That means not only depending upon yourself, but also not taking the direction of anyone else who says "you *must* do this" in terms of defining success and setting your goals and priorities. Of course, getting advice on both the process and content of the physical and athletic aspects of the *training and racing* endeavor, one of the principal functions of this conversation that we are having and will have throughout this book, is just fine. That's called coaching. But you must not mistake coaching for giving up *control* of your own *mental* approach to training and racing and why you are doing both. Taking control also means accepting responsibility for failure as well as for success.

Further Aspects of Using Your Mind
Ambivalence and Getting Ready to Quit

Even the most highly motivated, disciplined, and focused duathlete may feel like not training on a particular day, like not finishing a particular race, and even—in extreme cases—like dropping the whole enterprise. This feeling is called ambivalence. Ambivalence is a state of mind characterized by coexisting but conflicting feelings about a contemplated action, another person, or a situation in which one finds oneself. Feeling ambivalent is perfectly normal. Virtually everyone who even thinks about making a major change in his or her life experiences it—as does virtually every duathlete more than once during his or her career in the sport. I certainly have.

The key to success in dealing with ambivalence is to accept that it will always be present to some extent. Sometimes the ambivalent feelings will be weaker, sometimes stronger. What you do in response to the feelings determines their impact, determines whether they will trip you up, or not get in your way. If ambivalence destroys your commitment, that's a problem. If it simply *questions* your commitment, if it does nothing more than take you on a temporary detour, it can lead to a strengthening of resolve. Or it may be that you are facing a more serious roadblock, like an inner voice that questions whether you want to even begin or fears failure once you do get started. Do you hear yourself thinking any of the following?

I really don't want to do this.

I know I'll just never be able to get started.

I just know I don't have the time.

One day I want to and the next day I don't.

I don't think I have it in me to do this.

What do I suggest? In most cases, fighting the feelings doesn't work. Rather, go with the flow. If you really feel like stopping that training day, that race, that season, forever even (yes, I can say this), remember, that's OK, *if it works for you, if it is going to have some positive outcome.* That is the key. Does what you are doing do something positive for you? Unless you are an outstanding athlete who can consistently win in your age group or even overall, you are, or should be, in this primarily to have fun. Of course, winning, too, is great fun. I experience winning in my age group (or finishing second or third and still getting a plaque) on a fairly regular basis, usually when there are three or fewer of us in that age-group!

Still, when it stops being fun, it is time to stop doing it.

But then, maybe a "but then" comes along. You get up the next morning and say to yourself, "Did I really mean that? Do I really want to stop, for the week, for the month, for the rest of the season, or was I just having a bad race, or day, or training week?" And if you think, *Well, maybe I don't really mean quitting,* that's precisely when you want to go back to the Ordinary Mortals® Pathway to Mobilizing Motivation, perhaps this time stressing for yourself more than ever the element of realism.

Realism
To set goals that are going to work, the goals you set must be realistic, for you. There is a strong genetic component in

the determination of body shape and size. Similarly genetics can also determine whether you can significantly increase muscle bulk by lifting weights or whether you can achieve great speed as a runner. The goals you set for yourself should be suitable. If, for example, your body shape and metabolism have always placed you on the heavier end of the spectrum, a good weight-loss goal might be to become thinner rather than to become thin according to society's and the media's definition.

If you are not inherently fast, like me, don't worry yourself about placing in your age group. That is, unless you are prepared to spend a lot of time in speed training (and even that may not do the trick), or unless you are old enough so that in a given race there are three or fewer people in your age group and all you have to do to get an award is finish! (In my region, the New York metropolitan area, my age group has been a pretty small one since I was in my mid-60s; I was born in 1936.) Remember, going fast is the product of training *plus* natural ability. Many people (and I am one of them) simply will not be able to go very fast no matter how hard they try. To avoid frustration, injury, and quitting, you need to recognize that fact.

A good formulation of the "realism" concept is the phrase, "Gradual change leads to permanent changes," one of the Basic Eight of Regular Exercise. For example, after some reasonable stretch of training, say three to four months, many people will find that they can go quite a bit further/longer in their chosen activity than they could have conceived of going before they started. With that experience, Doin' the Du comes into view, or back into view, for many,

many people. In sum, whatever your goals are, knowing what they are and why you want to achieve them, and that they are reasonable ones for you, is absolutely central to achieving success in duathlon. Now let's move on to taking those first steps in achieving the goals you have set for yourself, finding and choosing your races.

CHAPTER 4

Finding and Choosing Your Races

On your mark! Get set! Go! The adrenaline is up! You're starting off on that first leg of your first duathlon. OK. Perhaps
not quite yet. But even if you are a first-time duathlete, even
before you begin your first Doin' the Du' Training Program
(DTDTP), you should be thinking about choosing your first
race. The information presented in this chapter will help you
find races and make a sensible first-race decision. If you are
already a recreational duathlete but have approached your
racing and race selection somewhat haphazardly, as you get
ready for your next event the information in this chapter
will help you get better organized. Whether you are a first-
timer or a some-timer, doing races that are right for you,
on a schedule that makes sense for who you are, will make
duathloning so much more fun than if you participate on a
set of whims.

If you are a first-timer, you want to make sure that you
will have enough time to get in the requisite training before
you find yourself at a starting line. If you are starting from
absolute scratch, you will likely need about six months to get
all of your training in. If you have already raced, you want
to have some spacing between events. At the same time, you
want to be able to stay in shape effectively and comfortably.

Another aspect of choosing races is whether or not you have any previous single distance-sport racing experience.

Among the race characteristics to consider when making your choice(s) are race types and lengths, the availability of races that are convenient in terms of your calendar and distance from home, and the nature of the course(s). This includes hills, heat, shade, transition-area characteristics, road surface, traffic, logistic support, spectator opportunities, and parking. Additionally you'll want to take into consideration the availability of overnight accommodation (if necessary), registration procedures such as applying and check-in, and overall, how much of a challenge you desire. In deciding, you need not check into every single detail provided in this chapter. But again, having an organized approach to choosing a race and preparing for it will vastly increase the chances that you will cross that finish line happily and healthily, however many races you have done.

Types of Races

As noted in chapter 1, a duathlon is a distance race in which you engage in two sports (in contrast with a triathlon, in which you engage in three). Most commonly, there are three segments in the event, as in its sibling triathlon, but sometimes there are only two. The planning and racing logistics are much simpler than they are for triathlon. The most common duathlon is a run-bike-run event. There are also duathlons in which the course goes off road (with which I have no experience). There are two other two-sport combinations, both of which involve swimming—the aquathlon (run-swim-run) and the aqua-velo (aqua-bike). I have done one of the former and two of the latter. But since this book is intended for the nonswimming multisport athlete, I do not cover them in this book.

As noted earlier, the usual distances for the run-bike-run events are 2 to 3 miles each for the run segments, and 10 to 15 miles for the bike. There are longer events however. As of 2010, the distances for the USA Triathlon Age-Group National Duathlon Championships were 5 kilometers, 40 kilometers and 5 kilometers. The International Triathlon Union Age-Group Worlds that year covered distances of 10 kilometers, 40 kilometers and 5 kilometers. Then, there is the International Powerman Series, with distances up to 10 kilometers, 150 kilometers and 30 kilometers at Zofingen in the Swiss Alps. But most US races are at the nice, (relatively) short distances. Of course, if you find that you like multisport racing, there will be plenty of opportunity to do longer races in the future.

We've got a fun race here. Of course, there is no swimming. Just as the swim spreads out the competitors in the triathlon, so does the first run spread them out in the run-bike-run duathlon. Thus, it is unlikely that there will be bike-traffic jams on the (often narrow) roads on which most duathlon bike races are held. And there is less likelihood that large numbers of competitors will be close enough to each other to be tempted to engage in "drafting" (riding close behind a cyclist to cut down on wind resistance), a practice that is intrinsic to bicycle racing, but is against the rules in most duathlons. An advantage of duathlon over triathlon is that you only have to wear one outfit, although on colder days in early spring or late fall, for the bike ride many people do put on a wind shell over whatever they have been wearing for the first run. Speaking of spring and fall, because there is no worry about water temperature, in many parts of the country the duathlon season is rather longer than the triathlon season.

Race Characteristics
Calendar
If you are a first-timer, you should pick the date of your first race so that you will not have to begin your training in cold, possibly snowy, weather. And I would advise choosing a first race that will likely not fall on an overwhelmingly hot day. Thus, in most parts of the United States and Canada, June (if you are ready to go right into the Doin' the Du Training Program) and September (if you will need to do the Foundation Program first) are good months for your duathlon debut. In the US South and Southwest, you could comfortably begin earlier or end later in the year. For other countries and parts of the world, of course, similar considerations apply.

Getting to the Race
For openers, it's a good idea to choose a race that's reasonably close to home, enough so that you can sleep in your own bed the night before. There's no need to add the complication and expense of getting overnight accommodations if you don't have to. At the same time, you don't want to have to get up

in the middle of the night in order to get to the starting line on time.

Let's say that the start time is 8:00 a.m. You should allow yourself at least one hour at the race site to check in, organize your stuff, attend to bodily functions, and so forth. You can learn about the local logistics and about how to get set up properly in the transition area at a somewhat relaxed pace. You will likely be nervous enough the first time (or even the second or third) without having to add to the stress with unnecessary rushing. I've been doing this a long time, but still got nervous before my 221st event, an aqua-bike duathlon at a venue that was new to me. For one thing, I was unaware of the somewhat complex race-site logistics and then was delayed getting to the transition area. I got to the starting line just in time. Allowing too much time is always better than allowing not enough. It all means that you will probably want to find a race that is within an hour or so driving time from your home. Then, if it takes you an hour or so to get up and out of the house (as it does me), you will need to arise no earlier than 4:30 a.m., hopefully closer to 5:00.

On the other hand, you may just find it more convenient to stay right in the race neighborhood the night before. In most locales, if you are willing to drive three to four hours to get to a race, and stay over the night before, you will have expanded your race choices considerably. Indeed, once you do get into the sport, you may well want to travel around a bit to different races, just for variety and adventure.

How to find accommodations for an away race? You can often get lists from the race director. You can also use the web, searching either "hotel" and the name of the nearest community, or going to a specific hotel chain's website and plugging in the town name. If you do plan to stay overnight, it is a good idea to book your reservations as early as possible, because each race's close-by and reasonable-cost hotels and motels tend to fill up first, and not all races are held in areas that feature large numbers of lodgings. Since you will have a bike with you, do ask if you can bring your bike into the room for the night. If you can get a room with direct entry from the parking area or on the first floor, that is a good idea.

If you get ambitious, you may decide to fly to a race in another part of the country. That is a grand adventure, indeed, and one I have undertaken on a number of occasions. It is, however, not cheap. On top of the usual costs of distant travel, you will need to buy or rent a bike carrying case for the plane (some local bike dealers have this item available for rent). You will never want to ship your bike on a plane just in a corrugated bike box. The risk of damage is simply too high.

You will pay an extra fee for transporting your bike, and those fees have become rather high. For certain races, bike shipping services are available. You can find out about them on the race websites, by searching on bike/bicycle shipping services, and/or inquiring at your bike dealer.

At the race locale, you will then need to rent a car (usually a station wagon or van) into which you can fit your encased bike. You may not have the opportunity to scope out the race course in advance, as you can do with one that is within reasonable driving distance of your home. You will need to learn how to pack and reassemble your bike (allow plenty of time for that), or have your bike shop and a bike shop near the race site do it for you (for a fee). Some folks, myself included, have full-size bikes that come apart in two pieces, plus the handlebars/stem and the wheels that will fit into an airline-legal suitcase-size box. (Mine is a Ritchie Breakaway.) However, choosing this option does mean buying another bike and then learning how to disassemble, pack, and assemble it. On the other hand, it also means that your rented car need only have a fold-down rear seat to accommodate your assembled bike, not a large bike box. Nevertheless, even with all of the extra logistics to take care of, the chances are that you will indeed have a grand adventure, just like I have had. All of this is obviously not recommended for first-timers or those who have done just a few races.

The Transition Area

Any multisport race is centered around what is called the "transition area." It is here that you place your bike on a bike rack and lay out your race stuff next to it on the ground. You will either loop the brake handles over the rack's horizontal bar or rest the horn (the front tip) of the saddle on it. Just check with a neighbor to see how they are doing it. At some races, you can choose your own bike rack, but the racks are usually numbered. In that case, you must set up at the assigned rack—and do so sometimes at a specific space—that is designated for your race number. You will place your biking and running gear on the ground to one side of your bike, laying it out in some order of use that makes sense to you. It's here that you will attach your race numbers to yourself and your bike.

You will usually find the starting line close to the transition area. For the sprint-distance duathlon, the overall race format is straightforward: first run: out-and-back, single loop, or laps; *transition area*: change to bike stuff; bike: single loop or laps; *transition area*: change back to run stuff; run: out-and-back, single loop, or laps; and finish. In almost all races, your finishing time is your total time from the start, time-in-transition included. If you are at all concerned about your overall time, how you set up your transition area space can have an important effect on your race time. Just make sure that the stuff that is out of your backpack or duffle bag and laid out on the ground is just what you need, and that *just* what you need is out of your bag. I do suggest bringing along some kind of ground cover to put your race stuff on, alongside your bike.

So, if you can find out about the characteristics of the race's transition area in advance, that can be helpful in making your choice(s) about which race(s) to enter. Hopefully, there will be plenty of parking, and the parking will be reasonably close to the transition area. This is not always the case, however. For example, my good friend Dan Honig's New York Triathlon Club runs three duathlons in Manhattan's Central Park every year. There is surely no parking provided for them!

Course Characteristics

There are a variety of course characteristics to consider when making your choice of race, whether it's your first or your fiftieth. In your mind, you should be comfortable with the course. If there is no anxiety about the nature of the course, then you have one less thing to compound the natural anxiety about racing.

If you can, you may want to find out about these course characteristics in advance: Are there any or many significant hills on the runs and/or the bike? Courses with uphills are not out of the question, especially on the bike leg because your bike should have a low-low ("granny") gear, what goes up must come down, and those downhills can be fun (except when the pavement is wet). But, especially for the first time, on the bike you would rather not encounter hills that are too long or too steep. And on the run, whether you are a beginner or an experienced duathlete, hills of any steepness are never fun going up, even if you know that you will be coming down the same hill.

If the race is going to be in hot weather, is there shade on either course or (hopefully) both? What kind of fluids availability is there at the transition area and out on the courses? What is the road surface like? Safety is, of course, important. You don't want run or bike courses that either cross themselves or each other (although I do believe that the days when such courses were set up are long in the past). Are the run and/or bike courses open to traffic? These days, if for no other reason than liability concern, an open-to-traffic course should have very good traffic control provided by a combination of police and race-volunteers.

Race Application and Registration

To enter a race, you will need to file a race application, sign a liability waiver, and pay the entry fee. Fees range from $20 to $100, but for most sprint-distance duathlons fees are in the $40 to $70 range (as of 2011). For many duathlons, you will need to apply through the mail or more commonly now on the web before the race. For some races, especially the longer and/or heavily attended ones, the day before the race you are required to confirm your participation at a registration area and pick up your race numbers, goodie bag, race T-shirt, and digital timing chip (see chapter 9). (The goodie bag will usually have an energy bar or gel pack or two, sometimes a souvenir and, almost always, ads for future races.) However, some races will still provide a morning-of-the-race application process, which is usually more expensive than early application, plus no free T-shirt(!), and may well require standing in a rather long line. Many races also have a separate morning-of-the-race registration for previously entered participants. Virtually every race now has a website with details of the registration procedures/requirements.

Competitor Support
It will help you to have a more enjoyable experience than you might otherwise if you can be certain in advance that the race is well organized, from registration to the provision of after-race food and the awards ceremony, that there is an adequate number of aid stations on both the bike and run courses, that traffic control is good, and safety on both the runs and the bike is a top priority of the race organizers. The best way to get this information is to talk with someone who has done the race before. Also, if you are bringing friends or family with you, you might want to check out the spectator opportunities.

Family Considerations
Speaking of family, there are family considerations in this sport. If you have a spouse or significant other, you don't

want to make that person into a duathlon widow(er). Bad news all around, from shortening your career in multisport racing to shortening the duration of your relationship. If your partner races, as well . . . great! But in many cases, you're the only one who does the du'.

Consider the following advice: In the standard, work-during-the-week/off-on-the-weekends family, try to stick with the training schedule and not pack your training into the weekends. The way the DTDTP is written, there are only a few Saturdays and Sundays on which the workout sessions last much more than an hour. You can do this sport without disappearing on the weekends. And try to work your during-the-week workouts into the standard family schedule as unobtrusively as possible.

As for the races, if you really get into it, try to pick most of your races such that you can reach them from home, without having to travel the day before (unless they are in really nice places that your partner would enjoy being in). If you are going to a race just for the day with your partner, think about making a stop on the way home to do something different that you both like to do together, like visiting a museum, or hitting the local galleries and shops, or having a late lunch at a special restaurant. If you travel together for the weekend to an away race, try to include some other non-racing activity like sightseeing in the local area or taking a walk in a local state or national park.

Watching a duathlon is not the most exciting activity in the world (even though doing it *is* exciting). In few races can spectators see more than the athletes leaving and entering the transition area and start/finish lines. And your contact with your partner during the race will usually be limited to a wave and a greeting here and there. So if your partner does go with you to the races, show lots of appreciation to him or her for doing that. At the same time, don't expect or attempt to require that your significant other come to every race. That way, the races your partner does come to will be more fun for both of you. For all of the above reasons and more, bringing small children to a duathlon is not a good idea, although there are some brave souls who do it. To be successful in this latter endeavor, both members of the couple have to be very secure in the relationship and with themselves and happy to accept the roles necessarily thrust upon them: One is the racer, the other primarily the caretaker for the children.

Finally, you can consider making racing a family affair. For example, if you have children who are old enough to race in youth duathlons and both spouses race, you could find an event where everybody can participate. There are also sprint-distance duathlon relays, where one partner does the runs, the other the bike. A really fun variant of that (technically a triathlon because it has three sports in it, but there is no swimming) is a race that my wife and I do every spring (our travel schedule permitting) in New York City's Central Park: the New York City Parks Department's Spring Couples Relay, run by Dan Honig. My wife, Chezna, does the first 2.2-mile run, I do the 12.4-mile bike (two loops around the park drive), and then we get in a rowboat provided by the Parks Department boat rental service on Central Park Lake, for a full loop on that body of water. I do the rowing and Chezna does the navigating. Great fun!

Finding the Races

There are a number of sources of information about available races. First of all, your local bike or running shoe pro shop will likely list at least some of the local races and may even sponsor them. There is an increasing number of triathlon/ duathlon shops in various parts of the country. They often sponsor a series of races and will certainly have lists for you. Many of the shops also have their own websites that carry race information. There are a large number of triathlon/ duathlon clubs around the country—for example, mine in the New York metropolitan area is Dan Honig's New York Triathlon Club (www.nytc.org). Dan's club happens to run about an equal number of sprint-distance duathlons and triathlons (mainly sprints, sometimes in conjunction with each other) throughout the racing season.

On the web, for a special focus on duathlon, you can consult www.duathlon.com/, a supporter of this book. You can find a national list of local triathlon/duathlon clubs put together by USA Triathlon at their website, www.usa triathlon.org/resources/for-clubs/find-a-club. *Triathlete* magazine (http://triathlon.competitor.com) periodically publishes race calendars and/or information about upcoming races. Independent websites also publish race calendars. You can find them, for example (as of 2011), at: www.trifind.com, www.trifind.net, www.race360.com/triathlon/races, www.calendar.slowtwitch.com, www.lin-mark.com, and www.beginnertriathlete.com.

USA Triathlon Sanctioning

Many duathlons are "sanctioned" by USA Triathlon (whose website was a significant source of information for this chapter). A sanctioned race is one that has, upon application, met the approval of USA-T. Sanctioned races meet the following standards:

The course is well-planned, and documented local permits have been obtained

- The event safety plan has been reviewed and approved by USAT staff.

- Proper comprehensive insurance coverage, including general liability and athlete excess medical, for the race sponsors, the athletes, and the volunteers is in place (and may be obtained through USAT).

- Professional USAT race officials, who are trained to ensure that each sanctioned event is safe and fair for competitors, are available to the race director.

- For adult duathlon races, the results will be scored in the annual USAT athlete national rankings.

- For sanctioned races (and the race application will tell you if a given race is sanctioned), you must either be a USAT annual member or pay a one-day USAT license fee. Just on the basis of the membership/license requirement, the break-even point for joining USAT (as of 2011) is three races per year. (Of course, there are numerous other benefits of USAT membership. You can find out about them on the website.)

A Final Thought

As you consult a race calendar, think about the list of defining characteristics discussed throughout this chapter and pick a race that's just right for you. Start your training program and stick with it. Don't try to go too fast in the race, and you will finish. When you do cross that finish line, be prepared to experience one of the all-time great feelings of your life. And if you're like many of us, you'll want to experience that high again and again. In that case, all you will need to do is go back to that race calendar and find the next race that's right for you!

CHAPTER 5

Getting Ready to Train

Let's say you're a first-timer. You're motivated, ready to go, all fired up. You're going to start training for your first duathlon. You want an approach that's going to work well for you, as a novice. Or let's say that you have already done a race or two, or more, but you're looking to develop a more organized, more time-efficient, more productive training regimen. As either a beginner or a sometime recreational duathlete, you know that you have to train. We've talked a bit about training in general terms. Now it's time to start down the road that's going to change your life—that is, it will if you stay on it. Get ready to train!

The Eight Principles of the DTDTP

Each element of the Doin' the Du Training Program (DTDTP) is based on precepts set down some years ago by the world-renowned running coach at the University of Oregon, Bill Bowerman. Coach Bowerman, who trained many of the top US middle-distance runners of his time, established ten principles for race preparation. The first seven of my eight principles of the DTDTP are adapted from his ten (the last is my contribution to it):

1. Training must be regular and consistent, according to a long-term plan.

2. The watchword is moderation.

3. The workload must be balanced, and overtraining must be avoided.

4. Goals should be clearly established. They must be understood, and they must be rational, realistic, and reasonable (the Three Rs).

5. Training schedules should be set up with a hard/ easy rotation, both from day to day and more generally over time.

6. Regular rest should be scheduled.

7. Whenever possible, working out should be fun.

8. Gradual change leads to permanent changes.

Let's take a look at them in order.

1. **Regularity.** The term "regularity" refers to the distribution of training sessions during the week and the distribution of workout weeks over the course of the racing season and the year. Both should be fairly even. It's a good idea to follow the suggested training-session plan fairly closely. For example, the maintenance (off-season) program (see chapter 6, table 6.3) provides for an average of three hours per week workout time. You could meet this requirement by working out for an hour on Saturday and two hours on

Sunday. However, this approach would benefit neither your musculoskeletal nor your cardiovascular conditioning nearly as much as a more regular distribution of shorter workouts. Furthermore, if your heart rate were to reach a really high level on the weekends only, which it might if you trained only then, you could, for example, significantly increase your risk of developing a serious heart problem during exercise. In addition, your muscles could be harmed by such an approach. Muscles worked out on a regular basis, on consecutive or alternate days, go through a cycle of buildup, breakdown, and further buildup, leading to increased strength and endurance. Intermittent workouts generally don't lead to the achievement of those ends. Pain and stiffness are the more likely outcomes of such an approach.

2. **Consistency.** Consistency refers to workout length. As indicated in each of the DTDTP components, I recommend that you not vary the length of time widely from one session to the next (for instance, training for fifteen minutes one day, an hour and a half the next). For reasons similar to those that militate against irregularity in training, inconsistency can interfere with the development of both musculoskeletal and cardiovascular fitness, and significantly increase the risk of injury and illness. As I write this book, I have been training regularly and consistently for my twenty-nine years in multisport racing. Doing so is a central element in making it possible for me to have stayed in the sport for so many years, especially since I didn't do my first triathlon until I was forty-six years old, my first duathlon until I was forty-seven.

3. **Moderation and Balance.** You should think of these throughout your training. Strive to stay in balance in the time you spend training, in the speeds at which you train, and in the difficulties of the course that you train on (hills and such). And don't overtrain. Training too much can become very wearing on your body and your mind. "Too much," of course, needs to be defined in terms of what your goals are and your present physical state and abilities. For example, let's say that once you get into the sport you decide to go for speed. At that point, what was too much when you were starting out might be just right once you are moving right along. Hey, you never know. (If you reach a point where you start to feel comfortable going faster and doing so appeals to you, you may want to look for a coach, a process we'll address later.) You will also be well advised to maintain balance in your life as a whole, in relation to your training and racing. Some years ago, triathlete Larry Kaiser of Cape Cod, Massachusetts, wrote to me saying, "I have always believed training should fill in the spare time of our days rather than consume our entire day or take time away from other important activities such as friends, family, work, other hobbies and relaxation." Balance in our lives, as well as in our training. I couldn't agree more.

4. **Goal Setting.** Setting rational, realistic, and reasonable goals (the three Rs), *achievable* goals, is central to being successful in the sport, with "success" defined by you, for you. And I'll suggest that having fun should be part of your definition of success.

5. and 6. Hard-Easy Rotation and Regular Rest. These two concepts are central features of the DTDTPs. Neither consistency nor regularity are interfered with by taking regularly scheduled rest. In my view, they are enhanced by regular rest. Note that days off are part of each training program, as is hard/easy, even as the length of your workouts is built up. If you're starting from scratch and have begun early enough in the season to be able to allow for a week off between completing the foundation program and commencing the sprint-distance program, and can still make your intended first race . . . do it! Certainly, after you've finished your season, even your first one, if you've trained consistently and regularly, take a week or two or even three off before beginning your maintenance program for the off-season. I always do. You'll give your body and your mind much-needed rest. And if you're a recreational duathlete already, a week's downtime at midseason has much to recommend it. Despite what you may have read elsewhere, unless you are front of the pack and completely in shape, while you'll lose a bit of your conditioning over a week or two, experience shows that you won't lose too much of it. And your mind and your body will be much the better off for the break.

7. Working Out Should Be Fun. Does this mean that you can expect to laugh your way through every workout? Does it mean that running and cycling will never hurt? Does it mean that every course you choose will be a piece of cake and on every training day the weather will be just right? No, no, and no. It does mean that you will be on a training program that has features 1 to 3 and 5 to 6 in it. It also means your training program will enable you to reach your goals (4). Almost every race I have done in my twenty-nine years in the sport has been fun for me for one or more of the following reasons: I crossed the finish line happily and healthily. I did a race I had never done before, so I had a new challenge. I did one of my "regulars," where I know every turn and every bump in the road, making things ever so comfy. There were three or fewer of us in my age group, so I came home with a plaque. I saw some friends who I see only at the races. Yet, I know how much I have to train to get to the starting line and then cross the finish line so that I can say, "Yes, for one or more of the reason above, I had fun in that race." Combine the two sentiments (and know that we all have days when it just plain isn't fun, in any sense) and you can say that either a) I *am* having fun working out, or b) I know that I *will* have fun in a given race because I have done my scheduled workouts.

8. **Gradual Change Leads to Permanent Changes.** Finally we come to the last principle. Because it has worked so well for me over many years, I like to repeat it on a regular basis. The description of the foundation program in the following chapter demonstrates in detail how the principle works. In short, starting gradually but consistently can produce permanent—and impressive—changes. My original Ordinary Mortals® triathlon training programs, on which the DTDTPs are based, rely on this important principle, which I first learned about from writer/coach Ardy Friedberg's *How to Run Your First Marathon* training program. His program required only twenty-four weeks for beginners to start from

scratch and end running a full marathon (at a reasonable speed). The training required was modest, averaging about four and a half hours per week for the last twelve weeks). It was used successfully by thousands of first-timers. Central to Ardy's approach, which I quickly adapted to mine, is the concept of "gradual change leads to permanent changes."

Medical Matters

Ordinarily, a normal, healthy adult does not need any special medical clearance to begin either the foundation or the sprint-distance training program. Each one begins with a fairly low level of regular exercise in terms of time and intensity. If you're going to experience any exercise-related health problems, you'll usually discover them early on, in most cases before you have a chance to get into real trouble.

However, it's always better to be on the safe side. So if you have any thoughts that you might have a disease or condition that would increase your risk of an adverse event if you were to exercise regularly at a level of some vigor, it's a good idea to be checked out by your physician before you begin training. If you have a history of any of the following diseases or conditions, you will definitely want to have a thorough medical evaluation before starting either one of the programs:

- Previous myocardial infarction (heart attack)

- Chest pain, pressure in the chest, or severe shortness of breath upon exertion

- Any history of pulmonary (lung) disease, especially what is called chronic obstructive pulmonary disease (COPD)

Any bone, joint, or other diseases or limitations affecting your muscles or skeletal system Further, if you have a history of any of the following conditions or lifestyle habits, having a thorough medical evaluation before starting either one of the programs is a good idea:

- High serum cholesterol

- Cigarette smoking

- Hypertension

- Abuse of drugs or alcohol

- Prescribed medication used on a regular basis

- Being overweight or severely underweight

- Any other chronic illness, such as diabetes

Now, if you do have one or more of the health conditions or problems listed above, you shouldn't necessarily be discouraged. Regular exercise happens to be useful in the management of a number of them. (It's also useful in managing certain dysfunctional psychological states, such as mild depression, mild anxiety, and low self-esteem.) If, following an evaluation, your regular physician or other health professional says "no," though you really feel the answer should be "yes," or if you've gotten an answer that doesn't quite seem to make sense, seek a second opinion. Not all health professionals know a great deal about regular exercise and its benefits for promoting health and managing illness, together what we now call "exercise medicine."

In many cases the key word for healthy exercising is "care." A person who is not entirely healthy may embark upon a program of regular exercise, *with care*. If you do have one or more of the above-listed diseases or conditions, and if you make the decision to go ahead, with or without consulting a health professional (the latter is not recommended), you should plan a slow, gradual, and careful beginning. Then, if you experience any increase in untoward symptoms characteristic of your underlying disease or condition, you should definitely and promptly seek a medical evaluation.

Cardiac Stress Testing

When I was starting out in multisport racing in 1983, certain exercise authorities recommended that virtually all persons embarking on regular exercise programs, especially programs as relatively vigorous as duathlon/triathlon training, first undergo cardiac stress testing. Now, according to the US Preventive Services Task Force of the US Department of Health and Human Services, there's no evidence that for an adult with no symptoms, getting an electrocardiogram (EKG), of either the resting or treadmill (cardiac stress-testing) variety, is either necessary or useful in reducing the risk of a negative outcome during regular exercise. The one exception to that rule is the group of males over the age of forty who have two or more risk factors for heart attack, such as elevated serum cholesterol, a history of cigarette smoking, hypertension, diabetes mellitus, being overweight, or a family history of early-onset heart disease. If you're in this group, having a cardiac stress test before starting to train for your first duathlon is a good idea.

A Final Thought on This Subject

If you've never exercised on a regular basis, or have done so only intermittently, or are a former regular exerciser who has been inactive for a year or more, even if you fit into none of the risk categories above, you should start with the Foundation Doin' the Du Training Program (see chapter 6, table 6.1). It is designed to enable you to reach a level of fitness from which you can then undertake the Sprint-Distance Doin' the Du Training Program with every expectation that you'll be able to complete it and finish your first race. As noted, it may not take you the full thirteen weeks to get to the point where you will feel comfortable starting the DTDTP, but it is better to get there too slowly than not get there at all because something untoward happens on the way.

Concerning Speed

Remember that speed is not just the result of how much training you do. But neither is it entirely preordained. Your performance in a given race is the product of both training and innate ability, as well as the weather conditions on that particular day. Some people are naturally fast and can do well in terms of finishing place without training too much. If they trained more, they could go even faster. But they're happy to not train that much and to simply go out there and enjoy themselves. Even though they are fast relative to many of their fellow duathletes, they consider themselves recreational duathletes. They know inside that they could go faster, but choose not to do the training that going faster would necessitate. On the other hand, if you'd like to train for speed and you think that you have the ability, I say go for it. In that case, you are best advised to use a designed-for-speed program. There are any number of books you can find to help you go fast, or at least faster (see chapter 12 for a few suggestions). You may also want to consider engaging a coach (see Choosing a Coach, below).

As for the naturally slower folks like me, you can increase your speed to some extent by training harder. I'm pretty slow, but, as you know by now, I accept my built-in slowness. As you also know by now, for me what counts is having been at the starting line so many times and crossing the finish line most of those times. I choose to get out there and enjoy myself rather than worry about my speed. And if on a given day I happen to go a little faster than expected, that's nice, too. Icing on the cake. But even for the naturally slow, if you want to get faster I suggest either getting that good book on speed training and using it at paces that work for you or engaging a coach who will work with you at those paces.

Aerobic Training

You've probably heard a lot about "aerobic exercise"—exercise intense enough to lead to a significant increase in the use by the muscles of breathed-in oxygen. The opposite kind—"non-aerobic exercise"—is that which is not so intense as to cause any significant increase in the use of breathed-in oxygen by the muscles. ("Anaerobic exercise," by the way, is intense, short-term exercise fueled not by breathed-in oxygen but by energy sources within your muscles.) Certainly, if you're planning to race with your heart rate in your aerobic range, you'll need to *train* with your heart rate in your aerobic range.

There is nothing written anywhere that says that if you're racing you must work out to an aerobic level of intensity. When you race at a sub-aerobic level, you're certainly not going to race competitively, but that doesn't mean you can't be there and have fun. Take me, for example. From how I feel, or from very occasionally taking my pulse during a race, or using a digital heart-rate monitor, I know that often in my workouts and my races, my heart rate is either not up in my aerobic range or it is at the lower end of it. But I don't primarily train my heart to go fast; I train my body and my mind to go (relatively) long. And I can do that without making my heart go too fast. If on a particular day that means that I'll be going fast enough to get my heart rate up into my aerobic range, fine. If not, that's fine, too. Nevertheless, I fully endorse aerobic exercise. For one thing, it has more long-term health benefits than nonaerobic exercise, And, as I previously noted, if winning or placing in your age group is what you want, that's going to be hard to do without training and racing aerobically.

How do you know if you're exercising aerobically? Many duathletes who are competing to win or place within their age group, and who perform well in those terms, both train and race using a heart-rate monitor that tells them just what their heart rate is. They need to get their heart rate well up into their aerobic range—how to find out your aerobic range will be covered shortly—in each of the three duathlon segments. The monitor will tell them if they're pushing themselves to their most efficient pace of that particular leg (see chapter 8 for information on heart rate monitors). Another way of determining your heart rate is by taking your pulse yourself.

Taking Your Pulse

We can't walk (or run or bike) around with little meters that tell us what our muscles are doing in the way of oxygen usage. But our heart rate provides a good and simple measure of whether or not exercise is aerobic. To determine your heart rate, you can buy a heart-rate monitor. Or, much more cheaply, you can take your own pulse.

You can do this at your wrist, but there's a much easier way. On each side of your neck there's a thick band of muscle that runs from the angle at the back of your lower jaw to the notch that marks the middle of your collarbone. On one side of your neck or the other feel with the index and middle fingers of your opposite-side hand along the front border of this muscle band. About halfway down, you'll come across the carotid artery, a large, pulsating blood vessel. You should be able to locate one carotid or the other fairly easily.

Caution: DO NOT DO THIS ON BOTH SIDES OF YOUR NECK SIMULTANEOUSLY. YOU COULD CAUSE YOURSELF TO PASS OUT, OR WORSE. Also, do not use this method if you have any suspicion that you might have carotid artery disease on even one side.

Once you've found your pulse, you can determine your heart rate with either a digital watch or one with a sweep second hand. Count the number of beats for six seconds. Multiply by ten and you have your heart rate per minute. That's all there is to it.

Exercising Aerobically

Various formulas have been developed for telling us whether a given heart rate means we're exercising at an aerobic level of intensity. In fact, there is a fair amount of academic controversy about the subject. Thus, while I present several formulas here, I am not endorsing any of them. A simple one that has been around for a long time goes as follows. First, subtract your age from the number 220. The resulting number is called your "theoretical" maximum heart rate, which is the approximate rate above which your heart simply cannot beat without sustaining damage in some way. Sixty percent of your theoretical maximum is now considered to be the minimum Target Heart Rate (THR) you need to reach to be sure that the exercise you're doing is aerobic. Table 5.1 shows the minimum THR for some sample ages. To be on the safe side, you should never exercise so hard that your heart rate goes very much above 80 percent of your theoretical max. A safe target zone is 60 to 80 percent of the number 220 minus your age.

Table 5.1				
Aerobic Heart Rate Chart				
(Maximum heart rate calculated at 220 minus your age in years)				
Age	Maximum HR	50%	75%	85%
20	200	100	150	170
25	195	98	146	166
30	190	95	142	161
35	185	93	138	157
Age	Maximum HR	50%	75%	85%

40	180	90	135	153
45	175	88	131	149
50	170	85	127	144
55	165	83	123	140
60	160	80	120	136
65	155	78	116	132
70	150	75	113	127
75	145	72	108	123
80	140	70	104	119
85	135	68	101	115

Knowing your target heart rate can help you pace yourself during aerobic exercise sessions. The heart rate chart above gives target heart rates based on percentage of maximum heart rate according to your age.

Aerobic exercise can be any activity that uses large muscles in continuous rhythmic motion to elevate your heart rate (such as rowing).

The American Heart Association (AHA) recommends aerobic activity for at least thirty minutes on most days of the week. According to AHA, target heart rate should be 50 percent of maximum for the first few weeks, building up to 75 percent gradually over a six-month period, then up to 85 percent. However, you don't have to exercise that hard to stay in shape.

There are more sophisticated formulas available. For example, some time ago Dr. Philip Maffetone, a coach and trainer for many top professional triathletes, recommended the 180 Formula. It produces one number for a recommended heart rate that, among other things, will likely reflect a level of muscle oxygen uptake that will lead to maximum body fat-burning for energy. With this formula, you first subtract your age from the number 180. Then, if you're recovering from a major illness or are on one or more major medications regularly, subtract ten; if you're starting from scratch, coming back from injury, or suffer frequently from colds or allergies, subtract five; if you've been working out aerobically for two years or less and are healthy, use the number as is; if you've been working out aerobically for two years or more, are healthy, and are getting faster/longer, add five. If you're unsure which of two categories you're in, choose the more conservative one. To arrive at a range for your workouts, subtract ten from whatever your 180 Formula number is.

Unmodified, this formula produces a number generally in the range of 75 to 80 percent of the earlier "theoretical maximum heart rate" standard (220 minus your age). The 180 Formula is more suited to multisport athletes aiming toward their eventual maximum potential. I find the range of 60 to 65 percent of 220-minus-my-age to be quite a comfortable zone for my workouts most of the time. That level of training brings me to a speed I'm happy with in most of my races, as you know by now. On the other hand, from the perspective of certain academic exercise physiologists, there is a wide range of variation and potential error when using either of the numerical formulas. Preferred is a qualitative measure called the Borg Rating of Perceived Exertion, or RPE (see table 5.2).

For some folks, qualitative measures of exercise intensity are perhaps as useful as heart-rate monitoring. If you're breathing reasonably hard, and/or sweating while working out in mild to cold temperatures, you can usually assume that you're exercising aerobically. There's also the talk test.

Table 5.2	
Borg Rating of Perceived Exertion	
6	No exertion at all
7	
(7.5)	Extremely light
8	
9	Very light
10	
11	Light
12	
13	Somewhat hard
14	
15	Hard (heavy)
16	
17	Very hard
18	
19	Extremely hard
20	Maximal exertion

9 corresponds to "very light" exercise. For a healthy person, it is like walking slowly at his or her own pace for some minutes

13 on the scale is "somewhat hard" exercise, but it still feels OK to continue.

17 "very hard" is very strenuous. A healthy person can still go on, but he or she really has to push him- or herself. It feels very heavy, and the person is very tired.

19 on the scale is an extremely strenuous exercise level. For most people this is the most strenuous exercise they have ever experienced.

www.cdc.gov/physicalactivity/everyone/measuring/exertion.html

© Gunnar Borg, 1970, 1985, 1994, 1998

If you can carry on a conversation with a partner (or yourself) while working out, you are, at least, not going too fast. Generally, meeting the talk test means that you are working out in the Borg scale at twelve to fourteen, which usually will correspond to being in your aerobic range. I can tell you from experience that heart-rate-monitor measurements and taking the talk test usually correspond for me. If you are working out at what feels like your top end, however, monitoring your pulse is a good idea.

On Coaching
What Is Coaching?
Coaching can be defined as an art and a science, the purpose of which is to provide advice, instruction, and motivation enhancement for both thought and action, with the primary objective of *improving or maximizing performance*, in the context of the person's goals. With these concepts in mind, you can then decide if you really need or want a coach. Coaching assumes that you have a level of ability in the activity/discipline, even if that ability is at the beginner level. The idea is to help you become better at what you are doing, with you first defining what "better" is for you.

Thinking about getting a coach? Well, multisport athletes at all levels can benefit from good coaching. USA Triathlon certifies professional multisport coaches at three levels of training, experience, and expertise. You can find coaches in your area by going to the USAT website and clicking on Resources. Of course, first you have to decide if you want or need a coach. That is, to come back to one of my favorite themes, you need to have clear in your mind what your goals are, what you want to get out of the sport. Do you want to go faster? For what purpose? To set a new personal record ("P.R.") or just for the fun of going faster, perhaps? Do you want to go longer? If you have been doing sprint-duathlons, is the goal to do that first longer one? Then, *why* do you want to do it? For yourself? (Good idea.) For someone else? (Not such a good idea.) Does setting such a goal elicit happy thoughts? Or are they more of the oh-my-gosh-why-do-I-keep-doing-this-to-myself type? Perhaps you want to improve technique without necessarily going either faster or longer (although better technique should equip you to do both). And again, why?

Choosing a Coach

Coaches come with a variety of skills, levels of knowledge, and attitudes. The most important characteristic that a coach for individual sports can have is the ability to understand and realistically assess a client; that is, he or she will have that central social-work skill of getting to where a client is. A good coach will say to a client, "What do *you* want to achieve? I will do my best to help you succeed in that." A good coach will help a client to define his or her goals real-istically, as well. They will not say, "This is what I think you should be going for." But based on what you say to them first, they will talk with you about what makes sense for you, in terms of your schedule, your health status, physical skills, conditioning level, and your natural abilities.

Then, if you are to be a good client, you will be able to talk to your coach about what you are getting—and not getting—out of the program as you move through it. Address any issues that arise directly with your coach. After all, you are paying the freight. If talking things out doesn't produce the desired results, change coaches. Coaching can be very helpful for many athletes at all levels of ability and motivation, as long as the right goals are set and the athlete and coach work *together* to achieve them in the right way.

Analyzing and Managing Pain

The recreational duathlete does not often have to put up with pain during a race, at least for any considerable period of time (unless the race is a very long one). But if pain does come, like Mark Allen, the great Hawaii Ironman champion of the 1990s told us he does throughout his races, you want to be able to manage it. You do that by using your mind. You get the pain under control, even adjust your speed to it: "I can take the pain that speeding up here will bring with it, because I do want to catch that rider in front of me." (Yes, even slow people like me from time to time will have a race within the race.) On the other hand, you might say to yourself, "It's OK, I can handle going a minute-a-mile slower on the run in terms of where I finish; it's going to hurt a lot less and that's worth it."

You will need to learn to know your body. Experience will tell you when the pain you are feeling at a given time during a training session or a race is from heavy muscle use, not from an injury. That kind of pain will go away in a few minute, when you finish or go on to the next race segment. Pain management is being able to act on that knowledge and keep going.

Several times in long races, on the bike segment I have experienced some knee pain or some back pain. I was able to deal with it because I had had it before, and I was pretty sure that it was just from exertion. I was almost certain that it would go away on the run, when I would be using different muscles. And indeed it did. So it was OK. The pain didn't worry me. It didn't cause me to become apprehensive of a possible future negative event. It just hurt, that's all. I went with it, managed it, because I knew what finishing meant, and I had mentally taken control of it.

On the other hand, if you experience a sudden pain or pain as a result of, let's say, tripping on the run or maximum exertion on the bike, that's something you should pay attention to, for that sort of pain may very well indicate an injury.

Now let's get on to the specifics of training for that race.

References

American College of Sports Medicine (ACSM), *ACSM Fitness Book*, 3rd ed. Champaign, IL: Human Kinetics, 2003. (I am a contributor.)

Friedberg, A. *How to Run Your First Marathon*. New York: Fireside/Simon & Schuster, 1982.

Jonas, S. and E. Phillips, *ACSM's Exercise Is Medicine: A Clinician's Guide to Exercise Prescription*. Philadelphia: Lippincott, Williams and Wilkins, 2009.

Maffetone, P. "Heart Rate Monitoring and the New 180 Formula." *Triathlete*, November 1994:10.

Walsh, C. *The Bowerman System*. Los Altos, CA: Tafnews Press, 1983.

CHAPTER 6

In Training

To get ready for the upcoming big race day, you will have to work out regularly and consistently, as we've discussed. And that will take a certain minimum number of weeks. But have no fear! In order simply to finish a sprint-distance duathlon, the total time you will need to spend in training won't be inordinate. You won't have to turn your life upside down to achieve your goal. At the same time, you can't just waltz up to the starting line and expect to get to the finish line, either.

Three Doin' the Du Training Program (DTDTP)* workout schedules are presented in this chapter: the Foundation, the Sprint-Distance, and the Maintenance. Each program is thirteen weeks in length. Recall that the sprint-distance duathlon usually consists of a 2- to 3-mile run, a 10- to 18-mile bike, and a second 2- to 3-mile run. Following the Sprint-Distance Doin' the Du Training Program" (see table 6.2) will prepare you for a race at that distance, assuming that you're already reasonably fit and working out regularly for two and a half to three hours per week. If you're not yet at that level, even if you're starting from scratch, in thirteen weeks the Foundation Doin' the Du Training Program (see table 6.1) will enable you to then start the sprint-distance program.

---

* Please note that the speed at which you can repeat those five letters, let us say ten times, has no bearing on the speeds that you will be able to achieve in your training and racing.

In the foundation program you average about two hours a week for thirteen weeks, finishing up doing three hours per week. This means that if you're starting from scratch and begin your training in March, you can expect to be racing by Labor Day. The Maintenance Doin' the Du Training Program (see table 6.3) will help you to stay in shape during the off-season. As noted, if you're already a multisport racer, but are training somewhat randomly and want to find a more focused, balanced approach to training than what you are presently doing, the sprint-distance program should work well for you, too.

Now, the hardier soul may move through the foundation program more quickly than I suggest and be ready to start the DTDTP after, say, nine weeks rather than thirteen. But as I first learned from Ardy Friedberg, author of *How to Run Your First Marathon*, and have had confirmed by many others over the years, it's a bad idea to go out for an hour, at full tilt, on that first day, or even on the fifth or the eighth, thinking that you will "get there" that much sooner. For most people, too much too soon is bound to lead to muscle pain, mental doubting (can I really do this?), perhaps injury, and an increased likelihood of quitting. *Gradual* increases in time spent, distance covered, and speed make up the proven formula for sticking with it and developing your body and mind for happy, healthy duathloning. If you *gradually* change your body's composition and athletic abilities, if you *gradually* change your mind's approach to what you are doing and why you are doing it, experience tells us that you are much more likely to make permanent the changes you achieve than if you try to rush either or both.

The Foundation Doin' the Du Training Program

All of the levels of the DTDTP are laid out in minutes, not miles. Their primary objective is to help you build up your physical and mental endurance, so that you can eventually be out on the course for the two to three hours that it will take the slower duathlete to finish a sprint-distance race. Obviously, the faster your training paces, the more miles you'll cover in your training, and the faster you'll be able to go in the race. But it is the total time spent, at speeds with which you are comfortable, regularly and consistently, that is the key to success with this training program.

Obviously, to do a duathlon, you need to be able to run and bike. But you don't have to be able to do both with complete proficiency in order to get started on the foundation program. If necessary, you can use some of your training sessions simply to become more proficient on the bike. In fact, you're well advised to spend the first four weeks or so of the foundation program just jogging or PaceWalking (my term for fast walking, which is described in chapter 7). That way, being a bit shaky in the more technical sport will not stand in the way of your beginning to develop your fitness, which should be your objective at this time in any case. Also, whatever sport(s) you are doing, let me emphasize the importance of easing into your training. Don't try to go too fast. Spend those first two to four weeks in the foundation program loosening up and in particular getting used to a routine of doing regular workouts. Later on there will be plenty of time to become more vigorous and technically rigorous.

Table 6.1							
The Ordinary Mortals® Foundation Doin' the Du Training Program							
Day	M	T	W	Th	F	S	Sun	Total Week
1	Off	20	Off	20	Off	20	30	90
2	Off	20	Off	25	Off	20	35	100
3	Off	20	Off	30	Off	25	35	110
4	Off	20	Off	25	Off	25	30	100
5	Off	20	Off	30	Off	25	35	110
6	Off	25	Off	30	Off	25	40	120
7	Off	20	Off	30	Off	25	35	110
8	Off	25	Off	30	Off	25	40	120
9	Off	25	Off	30	Off	35	40	130
10	Off	30	35	Off	30	Off	45	140
11	Off	35	30	Off	35	Off	50	150
12	Off	40	35	Off	40	Off	50	165
13	Off	40	35	Off	45	Off	60	180

Note: Times are minutes per day; 13-week total, 1,625 minutes; (125 minutes per week, average.

Notice that this program requires just four workouts on four separate days in any given week. The time spent in each of the workouts over the course of the program begins at twenty minutes in the first week and finishes off at sixty by the end. We are generally following the Bill Bowerman hard/easy principle here. By the time you finish the thirteen weeks, you'll be doing three hours per week, which is just below the weekly average for the sprint-distance program, and you'll have averaged just about two hours per week while getting there. Again, I suggest that you spend the first four weeks or so PaceWalking and jogging. At this point you will be just as concerned about getting regular exercise into your schedule as you will be about the exercise itself. So you should be doing something with which you are comfortable. As you add in cycling, perhaps beginning in week five, you can decide for yourself which workout sessions to devote to each sport. As you work up to it, I suggest eventually getting into a pattern of doing each sport at least twice a week. Since the workouts are all denominated in minutes, in terms of your overall conditioning, the sports are interchangeable.

Especially if you're just starting out, this is likely to be an exciting time of self-discovery. *Remember: gradual change leads to permanent changes; consistency and regularity are essential to success.* As long as you don't try to do too much too soon, you're going to enjoy the process, and you'll greatly diminish the likelihood of getting injured and/or frustrated. Enjoyment and staying healthy are the keys to getting to the next level. Stay focused on your goals, stick with the program, and you will get there.

Preparing to Race:
The Sprint-Distance Doin' the Du Training Program

You are now ready to begin the Sprint-Distance Doin' the Du Training Program. Remember that I suggest that for your first

Table 6.2							
The Ordinary Mortals® Sprint-Distance Doin' the Du Training Program							
Day	M	T	W	Th	F	S	Sun	Total Week
1	Off	40	Off	45	Off	55	60	200
2	Off	40	Off	45	Off	60	65	210
3	Off	45	Off	50	Off	65	65	225
4	Off	45	Off	55	Off	60	70	230
5	Off	50	Off	65	Off	60	60	235
6	Off	30	Off	25	Off	25	20	100
7	Off	25	Off	35	Off	35	50	145
8	Off	55	Off	65	Off	60	70	250
9	Off	55	Off	65	Off	80	75	275
10	Off	60	Off	70	Off	80	90*	300
11	Off	55	Off	65	Off	55	120*	295
12	Off	30	Off	50	Off	60	40	180
13	Off	40	25	20	Off	Race		

Note: Times are minutes per day; average of 3.5 hours per week for 13 weeks.

*These two workouts should be combined bike/run or walk workouts, so you can get some experience changing your clothing and doing two sports consecutively.

race as a beginner, and indeed for every race you enter as a recreational multisport athlete in the starting-out/getting-going phase, your goal should be simply to finish while having fun. As a recreational multisport racer, after you finish that first one—or two, or three or more—you may want to think about setting some reasonable time goal now and then, just to add some spice to the experience. But any time goal you set should be achievable through concentration and maintenance of a steady pace, without (figuratively or literally) killing yourself. The pace you wish to maintain in a race determines your training paces in preparation for that race. The idea is to train at a reasonable pace for a reasonable amount of time, calculated to make sure you're able to keep going on the course and achieve your primary goal of finishing, happily and healthily. That's what the DTDTP is all about.

Of course, in the sprint-distance program, it's the minutes, not the miles, that count. I hardly ever know how many miles I cover in training and don't often care. As in the foundation program, there are four workouts per week, spread over four of the seven days of the week: Tuesday, Thursday, Saturday, and Sunday. You can determine for yourself the best distribution of the two sports within your workout schedule, but for most folks two-and-two will probably work best. The number of minutes averages out to three and a half hours per week for thirteen weeks. The sprint-distance program is simply a reduced version of my original Triathloning for Ordinary Mortals® Training Program. The program has worked for me and many other multisport racers for season after season.

Should you use the Sprint-Distance Doin' the Du Training Program, get going, do one or more races, and then feel for one reason or another—you want to go faster, you want to work less hard during the race while staying comfortable, you want to do more races and make sure that your body can handle that—you can go to the Ordinary Mortals® Doin' the Du Training Program-Plus. It increases the amount of time you will spend training by about 35 percent, but is still very doable (and "duable.") In the amount of training time spent, it is close to my original Triathloning for Ordinary Mortals Training Program (TFOMTP), designed for what became the Olympic-distance triathlon (1.5-kilometer swim, 40-kilometer bike, 10-kilometer run).

Over the years, many a duathlete and triathlete has come up to me at a race to tell me that my original TFOMTP had worked very well for them. For example, I recall one particular first-time participant in the 1987 Seaside Triathlon (an Olympic-distance event at Hyannis, Massachusetts) who told me how helpful he found it. This might not have been notable except that he passed on this information during the race, as he slowly passed me by on the run leg. "Why did I have to be so helpful?" I thought at the time. Some years later the same thing happened on a bike leg, with the man passing me, passing on the information rather more quickly than the runner had.

More recently, I received the following e-mail at my university address:

"I just wanted to thank you for writing your book, *Triathloning for Ordinary Mortals®*. I'm a thirty-eight-year-old mother of two, and I never thought I would be able to say, 'I'm a triathlete.' But on Sunday, August 22, 2010, I finished the AFLAC IronGirl Sprint Triathlon in Columbia, Maryland. I finished in just under three hours and it was an incredibly

Table 6.3							
The Ordinary Mortals® Doin' the Du Training Program-Plus							
Day	M	T	W	Th	F	S	Sun	Total Week
1	Off	45	55	Off	55	70	65	290
2	Off	45	55	Off	55	80	75	310
3	Off	55	65	Off	60	80	75	335
4	Off	55	65	Off	60	80	75	335
5	Off	60	65	Off	75	80	70	350
6	Off	40	30	Off	35	35	35	175
7	Off	30	40	Off	45	45	55	215
8	Off	45	60	Off	55	70	60	290
9	Off	55	60	Off	65	90	75	345
10	Off	65	75	Off	75	90	90*	395
11	Off	65	60	Off	55	60	120*	360
12	Off	45	Off	60	Off	70	45	220
13	Off	20	20	20	20	Race		

Note: Times are in minutes; average of 4.75 hours per week for 13 weeks.

*These two workouts should be combined (bike/run or walk), so you can get some experience changing your clothing and doing two sports consecutively.

emotional moment when I crossed the finish line. It was your book that broke it down and made it possible for me. I came home to reread your book and get ready to start training for another triathlon. I can't wait to see if I can do this faster next year. Thank you again for sharing your knowledge and wisdom."

For my own training, if I am doing one or more Olympic-distance triathlons plus sprint-distance du's and tri's in my season, I use the TFOMTP. If I am doing only sprint du's and tri's, I use the DTDTP or the DTDTP-plus depending upon how many races I am doing (of course for me with swim workouts added for the tri's). Whichever one I'm on, once I've completed the first go-through, I generally repeat the week-six-through-week-eleven schedule. If I happen to be racing in any of those weeks, I count my race times toward my training totals. For sprint-distance duathlon training, that week-six-through-week-eleven schedule averages out to just under four hours per week. This will absolutely keep you in good trim for the racing season. If you want to make it a bit more rigorous, you can repeat just weeks eight to eleven, averaging just under five hours per week (more, respectively, with the DTDTP-plus).

Warming Up and Stretching

Stretching is a somewhat controversial area. Warming up is not. Virtually all exercise authorities recommend some kind of warm-up period at the beginning of each session before you go full throttle (whatever "full throttle" happens to mean for you), and some kind of cool-down at the end of it. A minimum of five to ten minutes of warm-up and three to five minutes of cool-down is a good idea. Once you're above twenty minutes per workout, whether or not you count those warm-up minutes as part of the scheduled time for that session is entirely up to you.

Stretching carries with it a number of benefits. The accumulation of research on it (as of 2011) has shown that among the benefits, however, are neither the prevention of injury nor of delayed muscle soreness (DOMS). Does this mean, then, that we shouldn't, or needn't, stretch? No. Stretching does increase muscle flexibility and joint range of motion. Of equal importance in my view is that stretching can make our bodies feel good. However, if stretching is going to do that, it has to be done the right way at the right time. It should also be noted that while stretching does not prevent injury, it can be very important in treating injury, when done under the supervision of a sports medicine specialist.

You should always warm up before stretching. You can stretch towards the beginning of a workout, during it, or after it is over, but don't start out stretching as the first thing you do. You should do stretches that are comfortable for you and work for you. The range of motion that you can achieve is what *you* can achieve, not what someone else can achieve with the same stretch. There are a variety of sources for finding stretches: books, websites, physical therapists, sports trainers, and watching at the gym. Just make sure that you get into it slowly and carefully.

In the Off-Season
Downtime

Let's finish up this chapter with some thoughts on winter or other off-season activities. First of all, I believe that everyone should take some downtime, some absolute rest, no training at all, during the year, usually at the end of the racing season. A week, two weeks, even a month if you've done a lot of racing, or perhaps had an injury or two that could use some plain old rest to help the healing process. As noted, if you're in good shape, you won't lose too much of your conditioning, even with extended rest. Many of the studies that show rapid loss of conditioning in the absence of training were done on people who had *just* gotten into shape. Research on well-conditioned athletes has shown that there's little harm in taking some downtime. The potential benefits of recharging the mind and the body are great. Some of the "positively addicted" distance athletes among us may find it hard to stop or stop completely. Irritability when not training regularly is a common complaint. If you count yourself among that group, and you don't want to stop completely, then at least cut back.

Goals Review

During the winter season, think about the goals you have set for your duathlon experience. What were the goals set for the past season? Were they rational, realistic, and reasonable ones (the Three Rs) for you? Did you have the mindset, the body conditioning, and the time availability such that your goals were achievable for you and where you are in your life? Did you achieve your goals, or at least some of them? If you did, did you feel good about it, did the effort work for you, or did you give up too much in other parts of your life and/ or get injured in the process? If you didn't reach your goals or did but didn't feel good, why not? Were the goals you set unrealistic, unreasonable? Did other things happen during the season that got in the way? How did you feel about that? How does your goal setting affect your feelings about your achievements or lack thereof?

The off-season is also the time to start thinking about your goals for next season. Do you want to do more races? Fewer? Do you want to do longer ones? Shorter ones? Do you want to try to go faster? Is it perhaps time to take a sabbatical? Whatever you do set as goals, continue to make sure that they're rational, realistic, and reasonable. As I've noted more than once, doing this sport should produce happiness, not pain. How you frame your goals can have a great deal of influence on both the mental and physical outcomes for *you*.

Off-Season Training

There are many ways to approach off-season* training. Some multisport athletes take off the winter completely. This is not recommended. Although you certainly can take off up to a month or so, if you shut down completely, next spring the road back will be a long one. At the other end of the spectrum are those who maintain a pretty full program throughout the winter. If you dress properly you can certainly run in cold weather. And you can bike, either indoors on a trainer of one kind or another, or outdoors if again you dress properly and don't mind having your feet converted into miniature icebergs.

But just as I don't recommend taking off completely, neither do I suggest just continuing your regular training.

---

* In most parts of the United States and Canada off-season means winter, when many of us do not want to go outside for our workouts. Of course there are significant sections of the US South and Southwest where that limitation does not exist. However, unless you are racing year-round (and for many of us that is not such a good idea in terms of the progressive accumulation of wear and tear on our bodies over the years), even if the weather outside is more delightful than frightful, I suggest making it an off-season anyway and changing your training routine.

Constant regular training never gives your body or your mind any rest. Your body needs some decrease in intensity to decrease the risk of injury. Your mind needs some of the same to decrease the risk of burnout. Thus, I suggest the happy-medium approach to winter training, the one I have used myself during my twenty-nine-plus seasons as a multi-sport athlete.

After your post-racing-season renewal period, get back into regular training, but at a reduced level. If you are doing sprint-distance duathlons, all you need to do in the off-season is work out for no more than two- to two-and-a-half hours per week. Next spring you will be able to comfortably get right back into the DTDTP. As far as winter training is concerned for myself, I've developed a cross-training program that involves some weight training, some abdominal work, some regular stretching, indoor biking, indoor rowing, PaceWalking (but only on dry surfaces), and some downhill skiing. I used to bike outdoors in the winter, but as I have gotten older, I have given that up. Too cold! I am not concerned about exercising aerobically during this time, just with staying active. I use the DTDTP Maintenance Program (see table 6.4), working out for a total of two-and-a-half hours per week (which happens to be the US Department of Health and Human Services rec-ommended minimum for health-promoting weekly physical activity). It keeps me fit, it keeps me sharp, but it doesn't wear me out over the winter. Come spring, I'm ready and rear-ing to go outdoors once again.

You can develop your own combination of activities, one that will work for you just as well, I'm sure. Just as long as you do something, regularly and consistently.

Table 6.4							
The Ordinary Mortals® Maintenance Doin' the Du Training Program							
Day	M	T	W	Th	F	S	Sun	Total Week
1	Off	30	Off	30	Off	20	30	110
2	Off	30	Off	25	Off	30	35	120
3	Off	30	Off	30	Off	35	35	130
4	Off	30	Off	30	Off	35	40	135
5	Off	30	Off	30	Off	35	45	140
6	Off	35	Off	30	Off	30	40	135
7	Off	35	Off	30	Off	35	40	140
8	Off	35	Off	30	Off	35	45	145
9	Off	40	Off	35	Off	35	50	160
10	Off	40	40	Off	45	Off	45	170
11	Off	45	40	Off	45	Off	60	190
12	Off	45	45	Off	45	Off	60	195
13	Off	40	35	Off	45	Off	60	180

Note: Times are in minutes per day; 13-week total, 1,950 minutes; 150 minutes per week, average.

One Size Does Not Fit All

Like me, many folks consult the sport magazines, various websites, and other sources for advice on training and racing. With all the information that's out there, how do you pick and choose advice? Here are some thoughts on how to go about answering that question. And the first answer is, very carefully.

So many of the articles that one sees regularly in the magazines have a one-size-fits-all approach. For example, take an article about strength training for cycling that appeared in 2010. It started off by saying "To make significant gains in on-bike strength and power, you need to be in the gym a minimum of three hours a week." Questions like the following don't appear: "Gains for what?" "Gains for whom?" "Why gain—do you really want/need to, for the riding you do?" Or, simply, how is "significant" defined and who is defining it, for whom? It then offers up a set of strength/resistance training exercises. One size fits all. Or how about an article on how to be a successful masters triathlete, offering advice on staying fast, competitive, and healthy over the age of forty. The article offered a singular approach to training with a major emphasis on speed. One size fits all. This is not to say that all such articles take this approach. Top triathlon coaches like Gale Bernhardt and Troy Jacobson make it clear at the beginning of their articles just who their intended audience is. Would that everyone did.

But let's say you're like me. As you know by now, I'm not fast and never have been. In my region, the New York metropolitan area, I regularly win or place in my age group only because my age cohort locally is small and getting smaller. Just because my age cohort is small and getting smaller I even qualify for the USA Triathlon Team USA and get to go to the International Triathlon Union Triathlon World Championships. (I don't take home any plaques there!) Of course I like to take home plaques from the local races, but I know that I get them not because I'm fast but simply because I've been in the sport such a long time and continue to show up! Plaques are the icing on the cake. My primary goal, the cake, is to have fun racing in eight to twelve tri's and du's each season, as I have done for just about every one of my twenty-eight previous ones. Thus when I see an article about staying with it and staying healthy, without being concerned with speed, that's one I will look at.

Just remember, when you are looking at the training and racing literature, one size does not fit all. You first need to know what your goals are. If they match up with the explicit or implicit goals set forth by the writer of the article, that's fine. If they don't, turn the page.

References

American College of Sports Medicine (ACSM), *ACSM Fitness Book,* 3rd ed. Champaign, IL: Human Kinetics, 2003. *Note:* I am a contributor.

Friedberg, A. *How to Run Your First Marathon.* New York: Fireside/Simon & Schuster, 1982.

Jonas, S. *Triathloning for Ordinary Mortals.* 2nd ed. New York: WW Norton, 2006.

Jonas, S. and E. Phillips. *ACSM's Exercise is Medicine: A Clinician's Guide to Exercise Prescription.* Philadelphia: Lippincott, Williams and Wilkins, 2009.

Maffetone, P. "Heart Rate Monitoring and the New 180 Formula." *Triathlete,* November 1994:10.

Walsh, C. *The Bowerman System.* Los Altos, CA: Tafnews Press, 1983.

CHAPTER 7

Technique

Good technique is important for the duathlon's two sports—the relatively simple sport of long-distance running, and the more complex one of cycling. However, to be able to finish a sprint-distance duathlon happily and healthily, you do not need surgically precise technique. And in my view you should not become centrally focused on technique, unless it becomes apparent that you have the potential to become competitive in multi-sport racing and want to do so. Becoming a technique fanatic may well take away from the fun and enjoyment of recreational duathloning, and might even get in the way of staying with it.

So, while we resist perfectionism, let's nonetheless spend some time on technique. It will be time well spent. Finding the happy medium, being able to perform the sports reasonably well without obsessing about it, is a good idea for several reasons. Good technique makes running and cycling more comfortable and more fun. Good technique decreases muscle pain while you are engaged in the activity, and the likelihood of getting an injury from it. It also enhances that feeling of being in control, which is oh-so-important to long-term success.

Further, good technique significantly increases your athletic efficiency. Take the following as an example: Have you ever seen someone riding a bike with the arches of their feet firmly planted on the pedals, and leaning far out to one side for one pedal stroke and then far out to the other side with the next? That person will get tired very quickly, unless he/she is in very, very good shape (or is a Tour-de-France competitor standing up on his or her pedals while going up one of those hills in the French Alps or Pyrenees). You generally want to have the balls of your feet on the pedals and you want to keep your upper body as quiet as you can. Also in cycling, learning how to select the proper gear at the proper time is very important. For example, to avoid getting caught going up a hill very slowly with your thighs burning, and being unable to shift down to a lower, easier gear because of the pressure on the gear-shift mechanism, you must learn to look ahead and down-shift to the lower gear before getting on the hill.

And so, let's move on to a consideration of technique for the two principal duathlon sports, running and cycling. After we consider running and cycling, we shall also look at exercise/sport walking technique a bit. Especially for those starting from scratch, exercise walking (which goes by a variety of names) can be a very helpful, useful sport in your workout program. Some people, myself included, also use it in the races from time to time, and not just when we are so dog tired on the run that we can't do anything else! Please note that I do not hold myself out as the expert on technique in any of the sports. For expert advice, consider consulting one or more of the sport-specific books listed in chapter 12, or a coach.

Running

One of the most popular sports for regular exercise, running is familiar to just about everyone. For most people starting, it is aerobic at all but the slowest speed. Running is cheap, time efficient, and readily accessible. You can run outdoors in most any kind of weather, and indoors too at health clubs and gyms that have tracks. (At the latter, running those short loops can become mind numbing if you are going any distance at all, however.) At home or in a health club you can also run on a treadmill (where the mind-numbingness can be relieved with a well-placed television set). By the way, you might ask what's the difference between running and jogging? The famous guru of running in the seventies and eighties, Dr. George Sheehan, said that the difference between a runner and a jogger is a race entry blank. Quite some time ago Covert Bailey, author of *The New Fit or Fat*, arbitrarily set a maximum of an eight-minutes-per-mile pace to define running. Anything slower than that was jogging, according to Mr. Bailey. I'm not sure where he got the number from. To my way of thinking, the best distinction is likely that found in the head of the athlete. If you think of yourself as a runner, then you are a runner, regardless of speed.

Running Safely

Running can be done over a long period of time without serious injury risk if done in moderation at a reasonable pace for no more than three to four hours per week, wearing shoes that fit and are in good condition. But people sometimes forget about moderation. They run for too long at too fast a pace. Or they are careless about the fit and condition of their shoes. If they then get injured, they tend to put the blame for their injury on the sport, not themselves. That is unfortunate.

Basic running technique is simple. Harold Schwab is a former national-class hurdler, who owns Second Wind, the running-shoe store that I frequent in East Setauket, New York. He once described running technique to me as "left, right, left, right." Well it's not quite *that* simple, but it's close. In addition to left, right, it is important to keep your body relaxed, bent forward very slightly from the hips (not the waist), back comfortably but not rigidly straight, head (and eyes) up, shoulders dropped, elbows comfortably bent but not locked, hands slightly below waist level as they pass your body, fingers lightly closed (fists not clenched), arms moving easily forward and back in rhythm with your legs.

You should try to keep your upper body quiet: no swaying from side to side or forward and back, no bouncing of the head or flailing of the arms. Extraneous upper-body motions just use energy unnecessarily and can interfere with forward progress. At the other end, make sure that you bend your ankles. Ankle rigidity can as easily lead to discomfort as upper-body rigidity.

For the foot strike, in the traditional method using running shoes, you land on your heel. However, you don't want to come down on your heel at a sharp angle, because doing so will actually throw you backwards with each step. Also, you want to take shorter rather than longer strides, again to avoid being pushed backwards on each landing. In two newer techniques you land either flat, but softly, on your midfoot, or on the ball of your foot. Midfoot landing is fairly easy to pick up. For on-the-ball landing technique, I would suggest seeking a good, up-to-date coach. They will be able to teach you how to do it fairly easily. (If you have used one technique for a long time and are considering switching to a different one, do so with caution. You could end up injuring yourself, experiencing leg pain of one kind or another.) In the traditional method, after you come down on your heel, you roll forward along the outside edge of the foot, and then spring forward off the ball of your foot into the next stride. If you are making a lot of noise with each foot strike, you are likely either landing overly hard on your heel or slapping your foot flat rather than smoothly landing on its full length, or leaping rather than gliding between steps, or taking strides that are too long. Overall, you should aim for balance, rhythm, and smoothness.

Stride Length
There is a significant variation in natural stride length from person to person. You may very well discover that yours changes during the course of a workout. You will likely take longer strides when you are going downhill, shorter ones when you are going uphill. When on level ground, you will find that if you make your stride shorter, you will be able to move your legs faster. Make certain not to overstride, that is, reach too far forward with your foot. That may look macho, but it will only lead to imbalance and possible injury, and could slow you down by creating a small braking action with each heel strike. Nor will taking longer strides get you through your workout any more quickly. Since DTDTP workouts are measured in minutes, not miles, you don't have to be in a hurry to get anywhere. By the same token, shorter steps will not mean a longer workout. Thus the right stride length for you is the one you are comfortable with, just as long as you are not uncomfortably overstriding.

Cycling

Cycling is an exhilarating sport, with a great deal of potential for expanding your sport horizons. Not only is it central to multisport racing, but you can also sightsee, tour, and commute on a bike. And of course there is bike racing, both on- and off-road, should you want to go in that direction at some time in the future. With proper technique, the risk of intrinsic injury is low.[*] However, its extrinsic injury risk is certainly much higher than that of running.[†] You do have to watch out for cars and trucks, pedestrians, dogs, potholes, runners, walkers both sport and casual, and other cyclists. Major attention to safety is a major consideration for any cyclist.

Top-form cycling technique is complex. It takes instruction, time, and practice to learn. To get you started safely and help you to ride effectively and efficiently at the beginner/recreational duathlete level, here are a few simple principles which will serve you well. Once you get into the sport, with some correct coaching you can become a high-tech rider if you choose to do so.

Pedaling

Most important in the realm of cycling technique is "cadence," the cyclists' term for pedal revolutions per minute (rpm). The most efficient way to ride your bike is using a high cadence

---

[*] Intrinsic injury is that which arises internally due to the nature of the sport itself; for example, cyclists' knee is due to overwork of the quadriceps (front-of-the-thigh) muscles, shin splints in running arise from the constant pounding of the sport, and swimmers' shoulder is due to the unnatural rotary motion.

[†] Extrinsic injury is that caused by a factor outside of the person and not specifically related to the athletic motion of the sport.

in a middling gear. As a beginner, you will want to pedal in the 60 to 70 rpm range on reasonably level surfaces. With experience, you will easily be able to work up your cadence to the 80 to 90 rpm range, called "spinning." Bike road racers usually try to stay in the 90 to 105 rpm range. Many practiced duathletes ride in the 80 to 90 rpm range, a generally comfortable one. But you might eventually find the higher, road-racing range more to your liking. Except when going up a really steep hill on which you cannot do otherwise, pedaling in a relatively high gear, at a cadence below fifty to sixty rpm, pushing a heavy load with your legs, is inviting knee problems. You should avoid it.

With each stroke, it is helpful to pull up to some extent on the pedal opposite to the one you are pushing down on. This will give you more power and share the workload between the muscles on the front of your thigh used in the push and those on the back used in the pull. If you use regular bike shoes with quick-release cleats of either the road or mountain variety (see chapter 8) you will find it fairly easy to pull up. You will also be able to do it to some extent if you bike with running shoes and a toe-clip-and-strap pedal (also see chapter 8). Both arrangements firmly attach your foot to the pedal so that you can pull up efficiently. (With the quick-release cleat it is much easier to disconnect from the pedal in an emergency than it is with the toe-clip-and-strap system.) In any case, except when you are going up a fairly steep hill, the "pull-up" is not pronounced. It is there to help with, not impede, the downstroke.

As with running, your upper body should be relaxed, not rigid, and as quiet as possible. Keeping your upper body quiet in cycling not only saves energy, but also reduces wind resistance. The only time when it is helpful to have a side-to-side movement is when you are going up a fairly steep hill, standing up on the pedals. Further, don't scrunch up your shoulders. That can easily lead to pain across your upper back. To help absorb road shock, your elbows should be comfortably bent.

Hand Position

Many beginning cyclists ride with their hands on the "tops," the crossbar part, of the handlebars. While riding that way is OK from time to time when handlebar control is not critical, the primary reason beginners do it is because that's where the auxiliary brake handles are on the cheaper road bikes. Using auxiliary brake handles on a road bike is not a good idea. If your bike has them, then you (or your friendly local bike mechanic) should get rid of them. Auxiliary brake handles have a soft, squishy feel. Thus, you really don't know how much brake pressure you are applying when you squeeze them. And if you have to stop suddenly, trying to decide whether to use the regular brake handles or the auxiliaries may lead to confusion. Confusion in sudden stops can lead to injury. I speak from experience. Many years ago, when I was starting out in the sport, I dislocated a shoulder because I got confused about which brake handles to use when going into a sudden stop. I ended up falling off the bike with one arm outstretched. Ouch! There was that shoulder dislocated. Once those auxiliaries are gone, you will easily become accustomed to using the main brake handles, mounted on what are called the "hoods" on the tops of the circular "drops" on the handlebars of a road bike, incorporated into the grips at the ends of the handlebars on a mountain bike.

On the road bike, there are two correct primary hand positions: on the brake handle hoods, and down on the drops, the outboard lower curved parts of the handlebars. As your speed increases on the bike, you are spending an increasing amount of your energy just moving air out of your way. Thus the lower you can get down over the handlebars, the more efficiently you will be riding. On long rides, it is important to change hand-position from time to time to avoid getting stiff. Getting a stiff neck from holding your head up so that you can see where you are going when riding on the drops is a particular problem to be avoided. (Oh yes, the recommended way to avoid that stiff neck is *not* to avoid looking where you are going, but rather to avoid staying on the drops for too long!) Hand position on a mountain bike is simple: out on the ends of the bars, where the grips are.

Changing Gears

You change gears on a bike by altering the configuration of the chain that, through the cog and gear arrangement, links the pedals with the rear driving wheel. You will notice that up front on both the mountain and road bike there are two or three toothed chain-rings mounted on a circular bracket to which the pedals are attached. Mounted on the right side of the rear wheel hub there are usually six to twelve smaller toothed rings called "cogs." The particular combination of front and rear rings around which the chain is looped determines the gear the bike is in at any one time. When the chain is on a large ring up front and a small one at the back, you are in a high gear. In high gear, requiring more effort, with each revolution of the pedals the wheels cover more ground than they do in a lower gear, and you go faster. Conversely, the combination of a relatively larger cog at the back and a smaller chain ring up front produces a low gear. Pedaling is much easier, but you don't go as fast. The lower gears are used when going uphill, the medium ones when on the flat, and the higher ones when going downhill.

On most modern road bikes the gear shift levers are integrally located with the brake handles. (You may still find an older quality used bike in excellent condition with the shifters mounted on the bike frame "down tube," the diagonal sloping piece that connects the handlebar tube to the pedal axle. It is perfectly usable, but the shifting is far less convenient than with the modern shifter-brake combinations. On some cheaper, and also generally older, road bikes, you may find the shift levers mounted at the center of the handlebars. Not recommended.) There are three major variants of the modern design (with shifter and brakes together) made respectively by the Japanese company Shimano, the Italian one Campagnolo, and the new kid on the block, the US SRAM. In each one the shifters work slightly differently. Your bike shop pro can show you the differences and instruct you in their use very easily.

On mountain bikes, the shift levers are generally mounted just inboard of the hand grips, either in front of or below the bars, moveable easily with the thumb without taking the hand off the bars. They also come in different combinations of up-shift/downshift keys/levers. Again, your bike shop pro will be very helpful in explaining the differences for you. Some mountain bikes have rotating collars on the inner portions of the hand-grips to control the derailleurs (see just below). Vroom, vroom! Just like a motorcycle, *nest-ce pas*?

You change gears by moving the shift levers or rotating the handlebar collars. Both devices are connected by wires to a pair of ingenious devices called "derailleurs." The derailleurs, one each for the front chain rings and the rear cog set, are able to move the chain laterally across the respective sets of toothed rings when you are turning the pedals and moving forward. Regardless of where they are mounted, on most bikes the two left-hand shift levers control the derailleur for the front chain ring, and the two right-hand shift levers control the derailleur for the rear cogs. For most shifting systems, moving the same little lever in one direction (usually toward the centerline of the bike) on the right-side shifter produces the opposite up- or downshift that moving the same little lever moved in the same direction does on the left-side shifter. (The SRAM system has just one little lever for each shifter. Your bike-shop person can easily show you how to use it.) It will take a bit of practice to instinctively know which lever movement produces which gear shift, up or down. Actually, it might take quite a bit of practice. After years of multisport racing, from time to time I still upshift when I mean to downshift, and vice-versa.

The beginner should bear in mind three important points about gear shifting: First, use the left shifter controlling the front chain rings if you want to make a major gear change. Use the right shifter controlling the rear cogs for smaller gear adjustments. Second, as I said at the outset of this chapter, when approaching a hill, be sure to drop your gear down *before* you start up. Otherwise, you may get caught in a gear that is too high for you to pedal in and not be able to downshift because of pressure on the chain. Third, don't be afraid (or embarrassed) to shift frequently. Doing so as you change from, say, a slight uphill to the flat to a slight downhill can help you to maintain that smooth cadence in the eighty- to ninety-rpm range that makes long-distance cycling fun and energy efficient. For more information on cycling technique, consult one of the books listed in chapter 12.

Walking

If you haven't been exercising at all, or have been doing it quite irregularly, and are planning to start out on the Foundation Doin' the Du Training Program described in chapter 5, it will be a very good idea to spend that first week or two in your workouts just walking in an ordinary way. Doing so will help you to start getting loosened up, and it will also help you to focus first on becoming regular in your workouts before you begin focusing on the two sports. Then you can move on to what I call "PaceWalking" for the next week or two (or three or four or more if you feel like it), before you proceed to running. (You may also decide to stick with PaceWalking at a good clip, that is Exercise PaceWalking, or use the PaceWalking race gait for the run legs of the duathlons. Both can be very comfortable.) Both ordinary walking and PaceWalking are perfectly legal gaits in duathlons (as well as triathlons).

Ordinary Walking

Ordinary walking is the motion of the body that, if physically able, we use as our primary means of getting around, one of those activities we all do with little if any consciousness of the motion. You put one foot in front of the other in a rhythmic fashion and you go from point A to point B. What differentiates walking from running is that when your front foot comes down, your rear foot hasn't lifted off the ground yet. In running, you are airborne for at least an instant between each step.

PaceWalking

PaceWalking is a form of fast walking using a defined technique that differs from that of ordinary walking. Fast walking goes by a wide variety of names: exercise walking, fitness walking, health walking, power walking, aerobic walking, sportwalking, striding. "PaceWalking" is a term I came up with some years ago when writing a book on walking for exercise. There are two PaceWalking gaits: exercise PaceWalking and the PaceWalking race gait. They are both easy to learn.

Exercise PaceWalking

In exercise PaceWalking you walk fast with a purposeful stride of medium length. With each step you land on your heel, feet pointing straight ahead as if you were straddling an imaginary white line, then roll forward along the outside of your foot, and push off from the ball of your foot into the next stride. As you push off, you should bend your toes up just about as far as they can go. Since you are walking, you will lift the toes of your rear foot off the ground only after the heel of your front foot has landed on it. Always having at least one foot in contact with the ground is what makes exercise PaceWalking a rather more gentle sport than running: there is much less downward pressure exerted with each foot strike.

As in running, you should stand comfortably straight, but not rigidly so. Your head should be up, shoulders dropped and relaxed. Muscle tension just leads to pain. Also, having your upper body nice and loose makes it easier to develop a smooth, rhythmic, comfortable, arm swing. As your speed picks up, you may find it more comfortable to bend forward slightly. That's fine. But make sure that you are bending from the hips, not at the waist, which inhibits full movement of your diaphragm, and interferes with efficient and effective breathing.

If you want to do exercise PaceWalking aerobically, the arm motion is as important as the leg motion is. If you are like most people, without a determined and constant, rhythmic swing of the arms, you will find it impossible to walk fast enough to get your heart rate up into your aerobic range. Your arm swing should be forward and back, in the direction you are moving, not across your chest. Doing the latter just interferes with your forward momentum. Your elbows should be comfortably bent. Swinging a straight arm often leads to the pooling of fluid in your hands. With the forward arm-swing, your hand should reach about to upper chest level. On the back-swing, you should stop when you feel your back shoulder muscles gently but firmly stretching. Your fingers should be closed lightly, your fists never clenched. Finally, your arm swing should follow the lead of your legs, not vice-versa. If you feel comfortable doing it, you can try rotating your hip forward with the forward motion of your same side leg. This feature will make your gait look something like that of racewalking (see below). But rotation of the hip is certainly not essential. Don't do it if it doesn't work for you.

Speed

As in all forward-motion sports, your potential top exercise PaceWalkingspeed is the product of natural ability, practice, and your fitness level. At the beginning, you will probably be doing about fifteen to eighteen minutes for the mile. (The average pace for ordinary walking is about twenty minutes per mile.) You can get down to thirteen to fourteen minutes per mile or even a bit faster with some practice. Should you want to walk faster than that, you will probably have to learn how to use the PaceWalking race gait or, for an even faster pace, learn how to race walk (see below).

Smoothness, Balance, Lift, and Rhythm

Smoothness, balance, lift, and rhythm are very important for an effective, comfortable, efficient exercise PaceWalking gait. As with running and cycling, you should strive to limit extraneous body movements as much as possible, especially in your upper body. Nothing herky jerky. As in running, the focus should be on moving ahead, not up and down or side to side.

The Racewalking Gait

Even with a hip rotation, exercise PaceWalking is different from racewalking, a fine but technically demanding sport. Racewalkers can move very fast, as fast as seven minutes per mile for more than 30 miles in the 50-kilometer racewalking marathon. (These folks are very impressive. I saw a racewalking marathon once, years ago. The racers were moving their legs so quickly that it looked as if they were floating just off the ground even though at any one time they always had at least one foot on the ground.) To get up to that speed, or even to eight to ten minutes per mile, requires a complex hip rotation that many people think "looks funny." Well, it is the most efficient way to walk even though it may look funny (at least until you get used to watching it). The hip rotation effectively lengthens the stride without overstretching the leg, and enables the attainment of much higher cadences than those of the ordinary walker or the PaceWalker.

Racewalking has strict rules: Of course one foot must always be in contact with the ground, and critically, the knee of the weight-bearing leg (right-left, right-left) must be straight for at least an instant each time as the body passes over it. This is hard to do without some practice. To make sure that entrants follow the rules in racewalking competitions, there are judges out on the course. Racewalking would be a very good gait for the recreational duathlete—fast, but with a significantly lowered foot pressure compared with running. However, I have rarely seen it used in multisport races. If you want to try it, you will likely need some hands-on instruction to get it right. In many parts of the country, there are racewalking clubs which should be able to provide instruction. As are all the other forms of walking, racewalking is perfectly legal in both duathlons and triathlons.

The PaceWalking Race Gait

Finally, in walking there is what I call the PaceWalking race gait. Essentially it is jogging while keeping your rear foot on the ground until you come down on your front foot. Even though it feels like running slowly, since one foot is always on the ground, you are—by definition—walking. Your knees are slightly bent through each stride, just as in running, and the arm swing is not at all emphasized. Your body is relaxed, bent forward slightly at the waist. With your arms, you just do whatever light, waist-level forward-and-back motion you need for balance and rhythm. As with exercise PaceWalking and running, you come down on your heel, roll forward along the outside of your foot, and push off from the ball of your foot. Your back is straight but not rigidly so, and your shoulders are relaxed. Your head is up, your gaze directed forward. A gait halfway between exercise PaceWalking and running, once you get the hang of the PaceWalking race gait (which can also be called "gentle jogging"), you may well find that you can comfortably maintain a pace of ten to twelve minutes per mile.

Try both PaceWalking gaits. You may really enjoy the sport. An increasing number of people are doing so. And if at the end of the second run leg in a race you catch up to some worn-out shufflers who went out too fast, you'll feel pretty good about racing with it too.

Weight Training

Some multisport athletes incorporate some sort of weight training in their workout schedule, especially in the winter off-season. I always enjoy working with weights, combined with some stretching and a sit-ups/crunches routine two or three times per week for three to four months during that time of the year. It fits in well when I have cut my running or PaceWalking back to perhaps once or twice a week on a nice, cool, crisp day. Although weight training is ordinarily used for developing musculoskeletal fitness rather than cardiovascular fitness, it can be done aerobically, whether with machines or free weights. It all depends upon the routine you use. Neither power lifters nor bodybuilders generally work out aerobically. Aiming for increased muscle strength and bulk, they are interested in lifting large amounts of weight for each "rep" (repetition) of the exercise in the "set" (the group of reps taken together), not necessarily in getting their heart rates up into the aerobic range. For them, the key is "high weight, low reps, low sets." They usually take a significant rest between each set, to allow the muscles time to recover.

However, lifting low weight with high reps in multiple sets, and taking little downtime between sets, can make the workout aerobic. At the same time, muscle flexibility and endurance, as well as strength to a certain extent, will be enhanced. You can lift weights at home or in a gym. For safety reasons, unless you have a partner at home, lifting with free weights (barbells and dumbbells) should be done only in a gym. And if you haven't lifted free weights before, you should be sure to get some instruction. If while lifting free weights you find yourself unable to support a given load, you might get seriously injured putting them down, or worse, dropping them. Lifting on single- or multistation machines can be safely done on your own. But even with a home machine, before you start you should get some instruction in using it. Indeed, if you are new to weight lifting, even if you are going to buy some weights and/or a home multistation gym (which can be quite expensive), it is a good idea to get at least a short-term membership at a health club/gym and pay for a few sessions with a certified trainer to learn how to do the sport safely. A modest amount of money spent that way could save you a major payout should you get injured from attempting to weight lift the wrong way.

Breathing

A final comment on an activity common to all of the duathlon sports. Breathing, as some experts like to tell us, is very important. Of course what they actually mean is *how* you breathe is very important. It is helpful to breathe rhythmically as well as to have a rhythmic gait, pedal, or stroke pattern. When breathing, you inhale oxygen, necessary for virtually every bodily function, but especially important to support vigorous exercise. You exhale carbon dioxide, a principal waste product of muscle activity. To get the maximum amount of oxygen in and clear the maximum amount of carbon dioxide out with each breath, you need to breathe deeply on a regular basis.

Deep breathing is accomplished by expanding your lungs outward using your chest/rib-cage muscles and expanding them downward using your diaphragm. (The diaphragm is the wide band of tissue that goes across the bottom of the lung cavity horizontally, separating it from the abdominal cavity. Moving it downward enables full lung expansion.) Deep, abdominal ("belly") breathing, fully using your diaphragm, is essential for effective carbon dioxide removal.

As your speed and breathing rate in any of the sports pick up, you will likely find that rhythmically linking your breathing with your steps or bike cadence will improve your performance. For example, you might breathe in for three paces, out for three paces. Of course, the right combination for you is the one that works for you. One exception to the "even, in/out" rhythmic breathing rule is a routine you can try when feeling suddenly worn out during a training session or a race. Exhale for longer and more forcefully than you inhale, say on a three-count-in/seven-count-out ratio, for two or three cycles. This is very effective in clearing carbon dioxide that has accumulated in the bottoms of your lungs' air sacs (the alveoli) because you are not breathing deeply enough. That accumulation often leads to a sudden "golly am I tired" feeling. The uneven breathing routine can be very effective in dealing with it.

Pity there is not such a simple routine for dealing with the fatigue you might feel on laying out the money for the equipment that you will need for duathlon racing. But hey, it's not as bad as all that. Take a deep breath, and let's go on to the next chapter—on equipment.

References
Bailey, C. *The New Fit or Fat.* Boston: Houghton Mifflin, 1991.

Jonas, S. and P. Radetsky. *PaceWalking: The Balanced Way to Aerobic Health.* New York: Crown, 1988.

CHAPTER 8

Equipment

Duathlon equipment and clothing come in three flavors: basic/vanilla, advanced/chocolate swirl, and exotic/simply heavenly cherry ambrosia crunch. In this chapter we shall spend most of our time on the basic, take a look at the advanced, and mention the exotic in passing here and there. For additional information, especially on the advanced and exotic stuff, you can consult the triathlon magazines or performance-focused books listed in chapter 12. In this chapter, the emphasis is on equipment and clothing for training. We will go over the specifics of clothing and equipment for the race itself in the next chapter.

Obviously, many of the items for training and racing are the same. But there are a variety of logistical matters that come up when you are doing a race, issues with which you are not concerned when training in a single sport on a given day. Those race-day logistics, too, will be covered in the next chapter. An entry-level set of duathlon clothing and equipment for training and racing, with costs in 2011 dollars, is presented at the end of this chapter.

Choosing the right equipment and equipping yourself properly is second only to learning good technique, for many of the same reasons. Good equipment makes the sports you are doing more comfortable and more fun. It also makes your activities safer in terms of reducing intrinsic and extrinsic injury risk. While working out, if you're comfortable and enjoying yourself and avoiding injury, you will significantly increase your chances of staying with the program. At the same time, just as it is not necessary to become overly technique oriented in order to enjoy duathlon racing, it is not necessary to buy top-of-the-line, expensive equipment at the outset (or ever). In any case, there is only one piece of duathlon racing equipment that can get to be truly costly—the bike.

Good equipment at moderate prices is available and it will certainly do to get you started. Depending upon your attitude, your budget, and what you want to get out of the sport, you may never have to upgrade that equipment. On the other hand, if you have the money and want to spend it, should you become a regular duathlete, there will be plenty of time and opportunity to for acquiring better-quality gear. If you are in the sport for years, like me you can end up with lots of fun stuff—and lots of extras and duplicates, too!

However, at the outset you may well be able to find much of what you need right in the "sports stuff" sections of your closet and dresser. Plus, you can start off with a bike from out in the garage or in the storage room down in your apartment or house basement. Heck, use one on a temporary loan from a friend or relative. The only other important items that you might not have, unless you are already a runner and/or cyclist, are a good pair of running shoes and for the bike, a helmet, bike shoes (if you are not going to use your running shoes on the bike [see below and the next chapter]), bike shorts and gloves. (Neither of the latter is a necessity, but with their built-in padding they certainly make cycling more comfortable!)

You can spend a lot of money on duathlon clothing, but you do not need to do so. If you cannot assemble a basic wardrobe from sports clothing you already own, you can put one together from scratch for $100 to $150 (see table 8.1) plus the cost of the running shoes, should you not already have a pair. Obviously, if you are comfortable running and cycling in a T-shirt, you can eliminate the running singlet and the bike jersey right off the bat. And so on, depending upon what you have and what your custom is, you should not have to spend too much to get started. Now let's turn to some specifics.

Running
Running Shoes

There are several characteristics shared by good shoes for any sport. First, the shoe must fit well, meaning that it touches your foot in as many places as possible, except over the toes. The toe box should be roomy—forward, sideways, and up and down. But otherwise your foot should fit snugly, so that it cannot move around inside the shoe, which could lead to blistering. In other words, a good sport shoe should fit your foot like a correctly sized glove with no fingers would fit your hand. And your heel should stay firmly down in the heel cup, not slide up and down within the shoe. No matter what, the shoe must be comfortable. Your foot should nowhere be squashed, pinched, or squeezed. Whether you are standing still or moving, the shoe should not cause any kind of muscle or joint pain. If you are a runner who overpronates (that is,

Table 8.1

Basic Equipment List (with prices)

GENERAL	
Warm-up suit, nylon or fleece	$75–$100
Waterproof digital watch	$25–$50
Subtotal	*$100–$150*
RUNNING	
Shoes	$60–$120
Shorts, liner shorts, singlets, T-shirts	$75–$100
Socks (four pair)	$15–$40
Sweatbands (two)	$12
Polypropylene long underwear (one set)	$35
Cap, woolen hat	$20
Athletic supporters, compression shorts, support bras	$15–$50
Subtotal	*$432–$677*
CYCLING	
Bicycle, good-quality, entry-level	$500–$1000
Bicycle computer, pumps (full-size and frame-fit), water bottles, gloves, other accessories	$100–$150
Bike helmet	$40–$200
Bike shirt, shorts, and socks	$75
Bike shoes (for clipless pedals) and pedals	$100–$500
Jacket, long-sleeve shirt, tights (for cool-weather training and racing)	$75–$150
Subtotal	*$890–$2,075*
Grand total	**$1,322–$2,752**

you roll your ankle in too far when you land on each step, a common problem) you should get shoes specifically designed to resist that motion. Overpronation is a common cause of injury farther up the leg. A knowledgeable running shoe salesperson will be able to tell you if you are an overpronator.

Running shoes are generally designed to provide good forefoot flexibility, heel cushioning, and heel support. For the heavier runner, there are shoes providing extra cushioning and support over the whole foot. For the overpronator, more resistive material is built into the shoe along its inside edge to help prevent that angling inward at the ankle that can be so harmful. There are also lighter shoes designed specifically for racing. But unless you are very light yourself, you should use such shoes only when racing. Generally, they don't provide the support required for regular training. However, if you really get into duathlon, they can be a boon on the run legs. As slow as I am, I do use them in the races.

If you have a particularly narrow or wide foot, you should try to find a shoe designed specifically to accommodate it, to avoid either having your foot slosh around inside the shoe or having it pinched or cramped. Some manufacturers have been known to make mostly wide shoes as their standard, but now most running shoe manufacturers supply shoes in different, labeled widths. Your running shoe store salesperson can advise you on that score.

To help prevent injury, it is very important to keep track of shoe wear. It can be tricky to figure out just when your shoe is gone. But it is better to discard a pair of shoes too soon rather than too late, that is, after you've got shin splints or pulled a calf muscle from using an overworn pair of shoes. In the better-quality running shoes, a telltale sign of overwear can often be found in the part of the shoe called the midsole. It runs the length of the shoe between the outsole tread and the bottom of the foot compartment. For comfort, midsole material must be somewhat compressible. As they are used, the midsoles in most running shoes will quickly develop little horizontal lines.

Take a look at those lines periodically. Too many of them mean that the midsole has become overcompressed. (Just what "too many" is you have to learn from experience, perhaps, with some help from your friendly running-shoe-store salesperson.) When that happens, the shoe is thrown out of balance. And so is your foot strike, possibly leading to injury, as noted above. Also, the wear at the heel of the tread is a good indicator of how worn the whole shoe is. If it starts to look run-down, have it checked out. Assuming that you have a good pair of shoes, if you are doing two to three hours of running per week, as a rule of thumb, after about three months of wear you should start looking at those midsoles. If there are many lines (or if the shoe appears to be developing a tilt to one side when looked at from the back) it is time to at least pay a visit to the running-shoe store to have them looked over.

Take your time when buying running shoes. Try on a number of different pair. Walk around the shop in them. Then, when you have narrowed your choice down to two or three, take each pair for a test trot in the store and possibly outside on the sidewalk if the store will permit you to do so, to see if they work for you at least in the short run.

Clothes for Running

As a general rule, clothing should be comfortable and—
except for support garments—loose fitting. To save time in
transition, top-level racers generally forego socks for both
the bike and the run. For the beginner and recreational racer
on the other hand, to help avoid blisters and just generally
have happier feet, it is a very good idea to wear socks. As for
clothing, there are modern fabrics, bright colors, and flatter-
ing styles available for both cycling and running. Some can
be fairly costly as athletic clothing goes. But when starting
out, it is best to spend your money just on the necessary
stuff that's offered at reasonable prices. Then, when you are
certain you are going to stick with the sport, you can wisely
spend money on that spiffy looking, latest-style garment you
saw down at the running-shoeor sporting goods store.

For running in warm to hot weather, you will need a T-shirt
or singlet (tank top), running shorts, socks, and running
shoes. Women will also need a sports bra and panties, and men
an athletic supporter. Possibly taking the place of the athletic
supporter or panties could be "compression" or liner shorts (I
always wear them). Also useful are a sweatband and, if you frequently run in direct sunlight, a cap and sunglasses. Further,
if you do a lot of running (and cycling for that matter) in the
direct sun you should use a good sunblock cream or spray on
the exposed areas of your skin. For running in cooler weather,
you may want to add a pair of tights, a long-sleeved shirt made
of one of the breathable synthetic materials, perhaps a nylon
or heavier running suit, a woolly cap, gloves, and an ear-
covering headband. (For more detail on cold-weather running,
see the section at the end of this chapter.)

Bicycling
Bicycles

While it is indeed possible to spend a great deal of money on a bike, you need not do so in order to enjoy the sport. Beginning at about $500 to $700 or so, you can buy a very nice bike of the road or mountain or hybrid variety that will give you many years of pleasure (see more on cost below). Formerly called the "ten-speed," the road bike is the one with the narrow tires and the curved handle-bars. The mountain, or all-terrain bike (ATB), is the one with the fatter tubing, the fatter, usually knobby, tires, and the flat handlebars. The hybrid has a frame similar to that of a mountain bike but is built of lighter tubing, with upright mountain-bike-like handlebars, and less-knobby tires, intermediate in width between those of a road bike and a mountain bike.

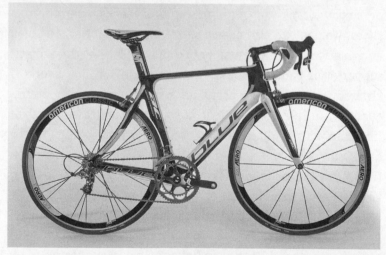

The classic road bike
Blue Competition Cycles/Steve Carrell

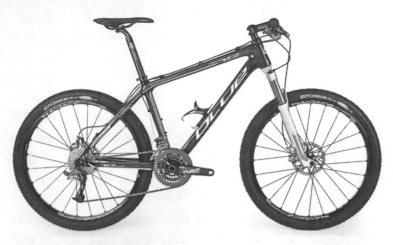

The classic mountain bike
Blue Competition Cycles/Steve Carrell

In most duathlons, you can use any of the three types of bike, but most mountain bikes are significantly heavier and significantly slower than most decent road bikes, while hybrids are somewhat heavier and slower than the road bikes. There are a few, mostly cold-weather road-course duathlons that require the use of the fat-tire bike, and there are the X-Terra duathlons, in which the bike leg is off the road, necessitating the use of a mountain or a cyclo-cross bike. The latter looks like a road bike, but has a higher road clearance, is somewhat heavier, and uses a tire that is somewhere between the road bike tire and the mountain bike tire in thickness.

Getting Started
The first bike for the newly minted duathlete is often that classic, "the bike in the garage or the basement" (or your friend's or relative's garage or basement). There are few

official rules governing the kinds of bikes allowed in duathlons. They must be person-powered and be propelled by use of the feet, not the hands. Other than that, you generally have your choice. (The use of recumbent bikes, while not explicitly excluded by the rules, is frowned upon as it would be in any bicycle race, for safety reasons. Actually, in my 220-plus races, I've never seen anyone on a recumbent.) Unless the race specifically calls for a mountain bike, you can use a road bike, or a mountain bike, or a hybrid. Again, don't be shy about using either of the latter if you don't have or don't like to ride a road bike. An increasing number of duathletes are doing so, and for the less-strong rider they can make those hilly courses much easier.

Just about any bike that meets the minimal rules will do. I have seen people get out there with an old Raleigh featuring a handlebar-mounted Sturmey-Archer three-speed gear shifter (I had one when I was a teenager, but it was long gone by the time I got into multisport racing); a touring bike with basket and luggage rack still attached; a local discount department store $149-special mountain bike (heavy as lead, but it goes); or that oldie-but-goodie Peugeot ten-speed that's been hanging around the back of the garage since you were in school (or after hanging around the back of *someone else's* garage for years, readily findable through the local classifieds or at a—yes!—garage sale). To get started, it doesn't much matter what you are riding on. If you like the sport and have the money, you will be going shopping for that first racing-dedicated bike soon enough. Or maybe someone will surprise you with one at holiday time or for your birthday! You never know. After a middle-aged friend of mine started out racing on his old Raleigh that he *had* kept since childhood, his children presented him with a spanking new road bike as a holiday gift.

Frames

When I started out thirty years ago, the top-end bikes had frames made of a chrome-molybdenum-steel alloy. The bike that I use when I travel by air to duathlons and triathlons, a Ritchie Breakaway, has a very comfortable, old-fashioned but relatively high-end steel-alloy frame. However, for the most part, this material is no longer used in any but the cheapest bikes. And so, when you go out to buy your first new bike for duathlon racing (or someone else goes out to buy one for you), for the most part you will be looking at bikes with frames made either of aluminum alloy (generally less expensive in relative terms) or carbon fiber (which range from more expensive to out-of-sight expensive—can you say $15,000 for a tri/duathlon-specific bicycle?!).

There are a number of design considerations to bear in mind. For your first bike, what are called the "seat and head-tube angles" of the frame should be in the seventy-three to seventy-four degree range. Lower numbers, found in outright touring bikes, provide a great deal of comfort and load-carrying capacity but limited responsiveness in steering, while bikes with higher numbers are generally stiffer and faster but can prove hard to control for beginners and even experienced recreational riders. You want a relatively light bike that handles easily and is responsive. It should also be relatively stiff, meaning that it transmits the power you are putting into the pedals into the rear, driving wheel, and not into flexing the frame, thus wasting your effort. Lightness and stiffness are important characteristics of a good bike, whether road, hybrid, or mountain. Of course, seeking the happy medium in this as in (almost) all things, you don't want a bike that's too stiff. It will give you a harsh ride.

Bicycle fit is very important, that is, appropriate frame size, proper seat height and forward-aft adjustment, proper length of the crank arms (the rods to which the pedals are attached), proper height and forward-aft adjustment of the handlebars, and so on. Over the past fifteen years or so, an increasing number of bicycle manufacturers have been making bikes with frames specifically designed for women. With the guidance of a good book chapter or bicycle magazine article on the subject, and with the assistance of a friend, given a correctly sized frame, you may be able to adjust the fit of your bike yourself. But to this day, given all of the variables listed above that should be taken into account, I prefer to have a pro in my bike shop do it.

Wheels and Tires

The wheels on a road bike should be 27 inches or 700 centimeters in diameter, two sizes that are very close in measurement, but slightly different, thus taking different size tires. (Mountain bikes come with 26- or 29-inch wheels.) Modern road bikes have European-style 700-centimeter tires with "Presta" air valves for the tubes. Hybrids and mountain bikes may have either Presta or the automobile-tire Schrader valves. To reduce wind resistance, the wheels should have thirty-two or fewer spokes rather than the usual thirty-six. There are also various kinds of high-tech, expensive wheels, constructed with many fewer spokes, or struts, or a disc. Consider them way down the line, if at all.

Modern wheels come in aluminum alloy or carbon fiber (again, expensive). Steel wheels may still be found on older bikes. They may sound as if they are tough, but because of their weight they provide a lot of excess rolling resistance. A good aluminum alloy or carbon fiber wheel will be as tough or tougher. (If you've got an older bike that you really like, one that has steel wheels, and you don't want to stretch for a new one, consider a simple upgrade to a moderately priced aluminum-alloy wheel set. It could make a real difference for you.) Light wheels require less effort to make them go around. Remember, weight at the outside of a circle is magnified by the centrifugal force created when the circle revolves. So a relatively small amount of extra weight in the wheel rims can make the bike significantly harder to push.

Unless you become a really good cyclist, you should stick with the standard clincher tire with a separate tube inside that can be replaced by a new one (or patched) if flatted. They are much cheaper and less finicky than the all-in-one tube-in-the-tire tubulars (also called "sew-ups" after their mode of manufacture) that are faster but only slightly so. When a tubular gets a flat, you have to replace the whole tire/tube combination. Once you know how to do it, changing a flatted tubular tire is easier and faster than changing a flatted clincher-tube. But learning the "once you know how" routine is not a snap: The replacement tubulars and the glue that holds them onto the rim have to be prepared beforehand, and there is the cost factor.

Cost

As noted above, you can buy a decent road or mountain bicycle beginning at $500 to $700 (2011 prices). If you cannot afford to spend at least close to that right now, and have or can borrow a serviceable bike to get started on, don't make a purchase. You may also be able to find a decent bike secondhand. But if you are a beginner, don't know too much about bikes, and do decide to buy a new (or decent secondhand used) one, it is better to pay a premium and buy from a bike store where the bike will have been vetted and serviced, rather than buying privately, especially if you don't know the seller.

Unless it is on a special sale, a new bike that costs much less than $500 or so won't be worth buying. It will likely have a lower-end frame and thus be relatively heavy, uncomfortable, and unresponsive. The wheels and tires are also likely to be heavy and thus offer a great deal of rolling resistance. The shift mechanisms may well be clunky and difficult to operate easily, especially on the hills. You will get a very good workout in terms of the effort that you have to put in to make the bike go. But you won't have much fun and will probably stop riding soon.

If you were to stick it out with a bike like that, you would soon be back in the bike store looking at the better bikes anyway. And then you might well end up with two new bikes, creating a serious storage problem, or a rationalization problem, or a "how-do-I-explain-this-to-my-spouse" problem. Owning five bikes, including two "number ones," a traveling bike, a cyclo-cross bike, and a hybrid, I speak from experience on this one. I happen to have plenty of storage space, but I have learned a lot about rationalizing and explaining to my wife!

If you can afford to go up to the $1,000 to 1,200 range, the significant difference in the quality of the frame and components over the entry-level bikes is usually worth the money. As to the more expensive bikes ($1,500 and up, way up) with sometimes weird-looking and sometimes conventionally shaped frames made of aluminum alloy, carbon fiber, or very occasionally now, fiberglass, and state-of-the-art components, wait on buying one of them, even if you can afford it. First see if you really like cycling and duathlon racing. Second, learn something about serious riding. If you have not done so, it is difficult to be able to feel, appreciate, and benefit from the features of the more expensive frames and component sets (and I speak from experience on this, too. I will never own a truly expensive bike—$5,000 and up—because I simply don't ride well enough to get out of it what it would have to offer me). Finally, regardless of how much money you are spending, it is a good idea to road test several bikes before you buy. If the bike store you have gone to demurs on that one, go to another.

Components

Once you get into buying a good bike you will hear the term "components." It refers to all the bits and pieces attached to the frame that make it into a bike, from the gear shifters, the chain, and the cogs to the handlebars and the seat. Like automobiles, bicycles are the product of the work of many hands and firms. The frame designer/builder is primary. But he can create a bicycle only by fitting onto the frame components made by a variety of other manufacturers.

You want a bike with the drive train (derailleurs, chain, and so forth), brakes, and the other essential elements basically integral to the frame (called the "gruppo," Italian for "group") coming from one components manufacturer. Thus you can be sure that the elements were designed to work together and will be of consistent quality for the price you are paying. As to all of the other pieces, bicycle manufacturers usually get them from different suppliers, but on the name-brand bikes, they will generally be of comparable quality to that of the gruppo.

Shifters and Gearing

These days, all aluminum-alloy and carbon-frame bikes come with indexed, click-stop shift mechanisms that make shifting gears much easier and more precise than the old gradual, slide-and-feel system you may remember from the ten-speed you rode as a kid (and may still have in the garage, not to say that you could not very well get started in duathlon with that old favorite). As to the gearing, don't start off with a racing cog set on the rear wheel. Be certain that you have at least one good and low granny gear back there to ensure that you will be able to get up hills while still on your bike. Rear-wheel cog sets are easy for a bike mechanic to change, so look into the matter of getting comfortable gearing on your brand new bike, even if it's a racing model. If you want to be sure of getting up virtually any hill that you might find on a course, you may want to have a triple chainring up front on the drivetrain. All mountain bikes and hybrids are tripled. You can now also get road bikes that are tripled, or you can change the usual double chainring to a triple at not much cost. (To my knowledge, I was one of the first to do this on a road-bike, back in the late 1990s.) Any pro bike shop worth its salt will be able to advise you on the proper cog-set selection and on a new bike. If a change is necessary they should make it for you at no charge.

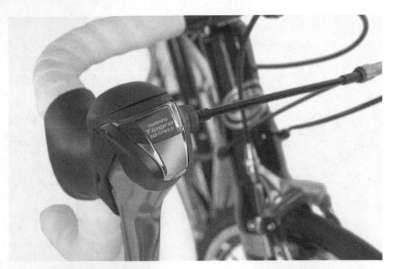

Typical gear shift lever
Blue Competition Cycles/Steve Carrell

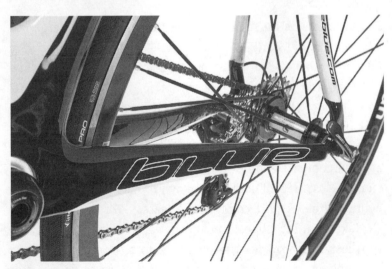

Typical rear cog set
Blue Competition Cycles/Steve Carrell

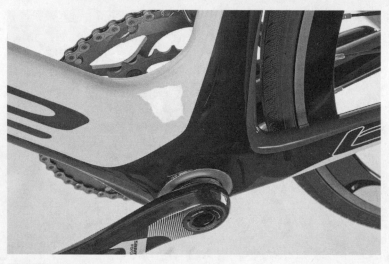

Typical chain ring
Blue Competition Cycles/Steve Carrell

Seats

The racing seats on some of the better road bikes are generally narrow and hard. They look great, but they can be very uncomfortable. If the bike you choose is equipped with one of those, and you would like to opt for a bit more comfort, don't be shy about asking for a good-quality, nicely padded seat in exchange. There are a variety of foam- or gel-padded seats on the market that give a very comfortable ride, but are still compact enough to provide the control you need for racing. Most decent and better-quality mountain bikes and hybrids already sport comfortable seats.

Like running shoes, the best seat is the one that fits you best and provides the most comfort. No seat will keep your bottom from getting sore forever, but some do a better

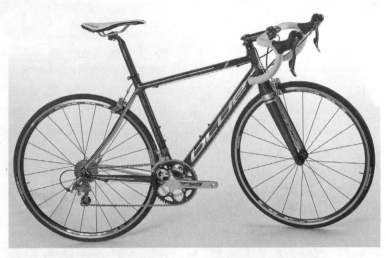

Typical racing seat
Blue Competition Cycles/Steve Carrell

job of it than other. Do not be fooled by appearance. Some uncomfortable-looking seats can be quite comfortable. So try out several, especially if you do not like the one that comes with the bike you have selected. Seats can be changed quite easily. In addition, putting a good lightweight pad/cover on a seat that is initially uncomfortable can help the fit and feel quite a bit.

As of 2011, the evidence purporting to show that bike riding causes impotence in men did not meet even the minimum biostatistical/epidemiological standards of validity. Nevertheless, if you find that one of the newer seats designed with the existence of your genitalia, male or female, in mind, is more comfortable for you, by all means get it.

Handlebars

Road-bike handlebars are of the conventional dropped vari-ety. Most people will find the handlebars that come stan-dard to be comfortable. But handlebars do come in different widths. If you think that you would be more comfortable with a different spread for your hands, that change can be made. However, since considerable labor is required to make the adjustment, it is unlikely that your bike shop will do it at no charge. I wouldn't consider going to a nonstandard handlebar width until I had quite a bit of experience cycling with a standard-width bar.

Then there are the modern du/triathlon-specific tri bikes that you will see at the better bike shops, equipped with aerobars. These are designed to bring your arms in towards the center of the bike, thus significantly decreasing wind

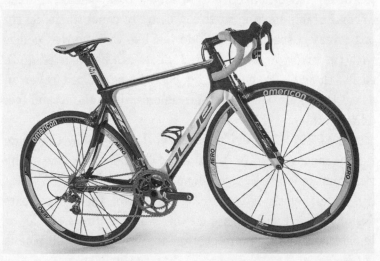

Typical road-bike handlebars
Blue Competition Cycles/Steve Carrell

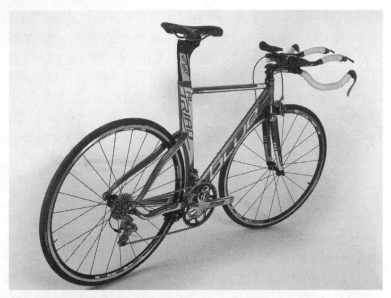

Typical "tri-bike" handlebars
Blue Competition Cycles/Steve Carrell

resistance. At a speed of 20 mph or more, over a 25-mile course, aerobars can save the rider around three minutes. That is nothing to sneeze at. At 20 mph, three minutes equals a mile. If one is competitive in one's age group, three minutes can easily mean the difference between finishing in the money or out of it.

However, at speeds less than 20 mph, the advantage does drop off. Furthermore, you may well find the bending over required for riding on aerobars and the tippy feeling that comes from riding in a narrow position to be rather uncomfortable. So, unless you think that you will be averaging 20-plus mph on the bike right off the bat, there is no reason to buy a tri bike for your first one. (You should not at any time consider installing aerobars on a road bike. The frame geometry of the latter is simply not designed for aerobars, and riding on such a bike would be particularly uncomfortable and unbalanced. I should know. Some years ago I tried it and rejected it fairly quickly.) I average 14 to 15 mph in the races. It would be much easier, safer, and less costly for me to pick up that time—let's say two minutes on a sprint-distance duathlon course—by speeding up my (notoriously slow) transitions rather than by riding a tri bike. So, as you have probably guessed by now, I do not ride on a tri bike. But that doesn't mean that you shouldn't eventually try one. At the appropriate time in your racing career, you might find the design very much to your liking.

And so, bottom line, my advice? Even though you might come to own a high-end tri bike one day if you've got the money and find that you are fast enough to make good use of it, certainly don't make one your first bike, even if you can afford the cost: a minimum of $2,500, more likely $4,000 to $5,000 (yes, you read those numbers right). Learn how to ride first. See if you are going to do duathlon racing for more than one season first. Objectively evaluate your ability first. And then think about the relative benefit to you of a tri bike versus a fine quality carbon-fiber road bike, such as the Blue Competition Cycles illustrated. There are many of those available in the $2,000 to $3,000 price range.

Cycling Shoes
While the shoe you wear for riding is obviously not the most important piece of equipment in the sport, it is important enough that I consider it a bike component, not a piece of bike

clothing. You can use your running shoes for a duathlon's bike leg as well as for the run legs. Many people do. But a running shoe is not an ideal cycling shoe. The principal characteristic of the cycling shoe is that it has a rigid sole. Its function is to keep your foot flat during the downstroke on the pedal. If on the downstroke your heel bends down from the ball of your foot, you lose power. Thus your pedaling will not be as effective if you bike with flexible-sole running shoes rather than with stiff-soled cycling shoes. Also, the width and tread design of the running shoe can sometimes make it a bit difficult to slip it in and out of the pedal toe-clip (see next section).

The classic road-bike shoe is that teardrop-shaped number that most people can't walk around in without feeling awkward. They used to come in any color you wanted as long as it was, like Henry Ford's Model-T, black. But now they come in as many colors as David's coat. That walking-around problem arises not only because of the full-length stiff sole, but also because of a protruding cleat under the ball of your foot that tilts you back on your heels. Nevertheless, they are the most comfortable, effective shoe when you are *on* the bike. If you get into serious, or even semiserious road-bike riding, you will eventually get a pair.

Mountain-bike shoes come with quick-release cleats that function like those on road-bike shoes (see next section). However, they are recessed into the sole, to permit somewhat easier walking. The quick-release cleat/pedal systems for mountain bikes and road bikes are not compatible with one another. Whatever shoes you buy for cycling, for your first pair at least, you should buy them only in a bike shop, from a knowledgeable sales person.

Shoe/Pedal Attachment Systems

The simplest attachment system is just the pressure of the bottom of your foot on the bike pedal. However, there is a great advantage, especially when you are going uphill, to having your shoed foot more directly connected with the pedal in some way, so that when pedaling you can pull up as well as push down. Once you try it for the first time, you will see what I mean.

There are two ways to make this attachment. One is to have a conventional flat bike pedal equipped with a toe clip. This device is a little cage that fits over the top of the pedal that you can tighten down onto the shoe by pulling on a strap that runs around its trailing edge, once you are underway and your shoe is firmly in the device. The simplest way to use the toe clip is to slide a running shoe into it. You don't get the advantages of the stiff bike-shoe sole. But assuming that the shoe's tread design doesn't hang it up on the pedal grid, you can get your foot out very quickly if need be. There are now several devices on the market that externally provide a stiff platform for a running shoe. You slide the whole shoe into it. They usually attach to the modern quick-release pedal (see below). Some duathletes are using such a device to save time in transition from run to bike and back again. But if a given device doesn't balance properly, it can be difficult to slip your running shoe into it.

The modern pedal system consists of a quick-release locking cleat that replaces the traditional pedal completely. It was developed to make riding with your shoes firmly attached to the pedals much easier and safer. Called "clipless" pedals, they have neither toe clips nor straps. There are several different systems on the market. But in any of them, a specially designed cleat on the bottom of the bike shoe snaps into or onto a spring-loaded matching clamp that replaces the traditional bike pedal. You snap out of it with a simple lateral movement of the foot. Once you become hooked on duathlon racing, more than likely you will find yourself hooked onto your bike via clipless pedals.

Clothes for Biking

Bike shorts are generally those tight-fitting black numbers with legs that extend down the thigh to just above the knee. Other colors are available, but basic black is the most commonly used one. Bike shorts come with padding in the crotch area. The padding used to be made from the skin of an alpine goatlike antelope called a "chamois" (pronounced *sham-wah* in French, *shammy* in English), and the material is itself called "chamois." Now there are a variety of synthetic materials available to fulfill that function, usually offering more cushioning than plain chamois. You can wear bike shorts as is, or with liner shorts (which is what I do). If the liner shorts are padded too, your comfort level will increase. Regardless of what you wear or do not wear with your bike shorts, you want to make sure that there are no seams in the crotch area that can cut into your skin in sensitive places.

Cycling shirts are usually called "jerseys" (the name originally given to a stretchy cloth made from the wool of sheep raised on the British Channel island of Jersey). They come in a wide variety of materials and colors. They are not essential for cycling, but they are comfortable and almost invariably come equipped with two or three pockets on the back that are useful for carrying items ranging from your house keys to your (light) lunch to a light jacket, in case you ride into a sudden shower. Bike socks are like running socks on the foot itself, but are cut low to end just above the top of the bike shoe. For wet, cool, and cold-weather riding, there are a variety of tights and jackets of various thicknesses and materials available. Bike gloves have open fingers, with extra thumb-protecting fabric and palm padding. They are highly recommended for rides of any length at all. The fabrics range from traditional leather with a webbed back to a wide variety of synthetics.

Other Bike Equipment
Helmets
The hard-shell helmet is the single most important piece of additional equipment that you will need for safety on your training rides and in the races and to meet the rules requirements, as well. It is simply not safe to ride a bike without a helmet. Eighty-five percent of all bicycle personal-injury-related deaths occur in cyclists not wearing a helmet. Serious head injuries occur close to ten times more frequently in riders without helmets than in riders with helmets. Simply put, you should never get on your bike without putting on your helmet first, not even if you are simply trying out a new pair of pedals in the street in front of your house. In the races you will be *required* to wear an approved helmet, with the chin strap fastened.

A decent one will cost you $40 to $50, although you can spend over $200 for a top-of-the-line model. Two important design characteristics to take into account when choosing a helmet, other than fit and comfort, of course, are coolness and weight. Generally, the cooler and lighter the helmet is (while still meeting the safety standards), the more expensive it will be.

All helmets sold have to meet minimum safety standards (see below). All multisport races, USA Triathlon sanctioned or not, for both liability and safety reasons, require that during the bike segment you wear a helmet with the chin strap securely fastened. The helmet must be of a hard-shell design and must have a user-adjustable or self-adjusting rear-retention system.

Helmet design has improved considerably over the years, providing both increased safety and increased comfort. Only helmets certified by the American National Standards Institute (ANSI), and/or the Federal Consumer Products Safety Commission (CPSC) are approved for use in any organized multisport race that I am aware of. (If you find a duathlon that does not require the use of a certified helmet, don't do it. That would mean both that their safety standards are low all around and that they simply don't carry liability insurance, which means you are on your own in case of an accident.) Certification is indicated by the presence of the certifying agency's sticker on the helmet headliner. Modern helmets should have either an ANSI or CPSC sticker or both inside. In any case, because of its own potential liability and required insurance, it is highly unlikely that an established bike shop or other sporting goods store would offer unapproved helmets for sale.

When buying a helmet, as with running shoes and bicycles, first and foremost you must make sure that the one you get fits you, and with the straps properly adjusted, is secure on your head. As to proper fit, it is important to make sure that the ear straps on the helmet are properly adjusted so that it cannot slip off your head should you fall and that you wear the helmet down over your forehead, sitting just above the tops of your ears. It should not be perched on the top or back of your head where it may be cool (in both senses) but can do you little good in a fall. You should adjust the chin strap as tightly as comfort allows. Your pro bike shop personnel will be able to advise you on proper fit and help you make the appropriate adjustments.

A couple of words of caution in buying, maintaining, and using your helmet. If it hits the ground with your head in it, microfractures can occur in the interior foam protective material or the hard shell, and the latter can tear. Thus, never buy a used helmet (for you cannot be certain of its history) and always replace a helmet that has hit the ground even once with your head in it. Further, the industry now advises that helmets be replaced every three years, for the protective material can dry out a bit and become less resilient. There are, of course, other factors which could cause you to buy a new helmet (or new clothing, gloves, or almost any other piece of equipment for that matter):

You've become such a good rider that your head has swelled and the old helmet just doesn't fit.

Your spouse insists it's time for a new color.

Your riding partners tell you it's time to get into the current era style-wise.

You can't think of anything else new to buy for the upcoming season.

Glasses

If you don't wear prescription glasses, using nonprescription sunglasses, plain or fancy, is a good idea for eye protection when riding, if nothing else. There are lightweight bike goggles/sunglasses for which you can get prescription inserts. I have used such an eye-protector for years.

Water Bottles

Water bottles are made of polyethylene or similar material and have a closeable nipple on the top. You can open the nipple by pulling on it with your teeth, so that you can drink while riding, holding the bottle in one hand. Bike water bottles come in two sizes, regular and large. You will pick the size depending upon how hot it is, how far you are going, and so forth. I will generally use one regular-size water bottle every ten miles or so on a warm to hot day. You will quickly find out what works for you.

Any decent bike comes with the proper attachments, usually two, for a water bottle carrier, called a "cage." If you are going to ride for any distance at all (more than thirty minutes), it is a good idea to carry at least one water bottle. With the wind in your face, it is easy to become dehydrated on a bike, even when it is not too hot. And you should get into the habit of drinking regularly, before you get thirsty.

Computers

There are a variety of small bike computers that will tell you your speed, distance, elapsed time, and in some cases cadence (pedal revolutions per minute), as well as, depending upon the design, other pieces of information. The information that the computer needs to make its calculations is passed to it by one or more sensors fitted to the bike at strategic locations. The sensors may be connected to the computer by wire (most common) or remotely using weak radio waves. There are also computers that have an electronic heart rate monitor built in, at added cost. Computers are generally priced in the $25 to $150 range. You can spend up to $600-plus for a super-fancy bike computer with a built-in GPS.

Repair Kit and Tools

If you know how to fix a flat on the road, you will then want to carry a portable air pump and a spare tube and/or patch kit. You can learn how to change a flat bike tire tube by reading about how to do it, but there's nothing like a hands-on lesson from your local bike-store mechanic. Unless you are into really high-performance cycling, you should look into installing Kevlar-belted tires. They are highly flat resistant. (These, too, I have used for years, with generally good results, even though they may slow you down a bit.) You might want to consider carrying a small CO_2 cylinder for instant inflation of a tube newly installed on the road. In the past couple of years, an inflator/"goo" device has become available. Once the cause of the flat has been taken care of (like pulling a nail out of the tire), with one of these you may well be able to fix the flat without even taking the tire off your bike. The spare tube, patch kit, the miniature tire irons you will need to change a flat, CO_2 cylinder or inflator/goo device, and a useful multipurpose folding bike tool can be carried in a neat pouch designed to fit under the bike seat.

You will definitely want to have a floor-model air pump at home with a pressure gauge attached. It is important to keep your tires fully inflated, pumping to the recommended pressure that you will find in text molded into the side tire casing at least for every other ride. (That text, printed or embossed on one side of the tire or the other, is not always easy to find and/or read. Using a flashlight can help to find it.) Among other things, this will avoid the pinch flats that can occur when an underinflated tire hits a bump and a small piece of the tube gets caught under the inside rim of the wheel as it flexes.

All of these accessories from tools to a modest computer can be purchased for about $200, including installation for those bits and pieces which need to be installed.

Bike Transport Equipment
Bike Racks
If you are driving to a race, you will need either a vehicle into which you can load your bike (and some people somehow manage to shoehorn bikes into very small spaces in cars) or you will need a bike rack. Back racks are available both for the car roof and for the rear (mounted on the trunk of a sedan, the lift-back of a three- or five-door car, or the tailgate of a sport-utility vehicle or stationwagon, or on a trailer hitch). The former provides a more secure ride for your bike(s), but is more expensive, and needs to be installed permanently (at least for the season) because of the cumbersomeness of the installation. The latter is cheaper and can be mounted just for each race to which your travel, but your bikes are hanging out there. A good roof rack will

run $200 and up but can be adapted to other uses, such as carrying skis or surfboards, as well. Rear-mounted racks run in the $100 to $500 range.

Indoor Trainers

Indoor trainers allow you to ride your bike year-round, switching from the outdoors to inside when cold weather comes. That does not necessarily mean that you will never ride outdoors in cold weather, on a clear, crisp day when the roads are dry. (Properly dressed you can have great fun doing that.) It does mean that you can continue to ride your bike regardless of weather and road conditions.

Riding indoors is accomplished by mounting your road bike on a device called an indoor trainer. The important features of this device are that it clamps the bike firmly in place and provides a smooth, adjustable resistance when you pedal. To vary the resistance you can change gears on your bike as well. Indoor trainers range in price from about $100 up to the $1,500 range for one that can be connected to simulated-ride computer programs or has them built in. If you already own a road bike and want to ride indoors in the winter, a reasonably priced trainer is obviously the least-expensive solution (rather than buying an exercise bike). You just bring your bike indoors and mount it securely on the trainer, and you are ready to ride. One fun way to ride indoors is to set up your bike in front of a television set or equip it with a reading stand. However, if you do either one, you have to remember to keep your cadence up while pedaling or you won't get too much from your workout.

Personal Electronics
Stopwatch/Chronometer

To time your workouts, check your heart rate, and—if you are cycling and don't have a computer—count your cadence, it will be very helpful to have a stopwatch. You can buy a good digital watch for $15 to $50. The most important characteristic to look for is that you should not be required to have a degree in mechanical engineering to set and use the thing. Also, the buttons that you press to operate the stopwatch function should "fall readily to hand" (or finger), as they liked to say many years ago in the British motor magazines.

You do not need a watch that is waterproof down to a depth of three hundred meters. You will not be anywhere near the water if you are duathloning. But a modicum of waterproofing is nice, say to fifty feet. Then, should you get caught out or purposely go out in the rain, you don't have to worry. By the way, running or PaceWalking in a light rain on a warm summer's day can be an absolutely delightful experience. However, don't go out in the wet on your road bike. Too dangerous. Mountain bikes are designed for the stuff, of course. If you are planning to do any nighttime training (foot sports only, reflector vest required), having a light in your stopwatch is very helpful.

Heart-Rate Monitor

This is a piece of equipment for the more serious trainer/racer. By telling you what your heart rate is at any time, it tells you just how hard you are working at that time. The heart-rate monitor consists of a lightweight belt that goes around your chest, containing a cardiac electrical-impulse sensing device and a small radio transmitter that sends a signal to a receiver/computer/display unit that looks like a large wristwatch. Some of the more expensive models have a stopwatch built in. You can even get them with a GPS, to (very) accurately measure your distance and speed.

Like many other accessories we have talked about, heart-rate monitors come in varying levels of complexity and expense (ranging in price from under $100 to more than $400.) The least expensive just tells you what your heart rate is. The most expensive provides and stores all kinds of information about your heart rate during a workout and can be connected to a computer for intensive analysis of the data. The manual that comes with the monitor will tell you how to use it.

An Added Note on Clothing:
Winter Duathlon Workouts

For cold-weather exercise outdoors, you should wear several layers of light- to moderate-weight garments rather than one heavier-weight set. Above all, you want clothing that is able to breathe, or let out through the fabric the moisture that accumulates as you get warm and sweat. Old-fashioned, heavy, cotton sweats cannot breathe in this sense. They just keep all that moisture in. Then, as it condenses into water and falls onto your skin underneath those sweats, it will make you feel colder, not warmer.

When starting out on a chilly day, you should wear just enough clothing to feel just a bit on the chilly side yourself. You are sure to feel hot and uncomfortable well before you finish your workout if on a cold day you feel nice and toasty warm at the beginning of it. No matter how cold it is, once you get going for a bit, you will begin to perspire.

Polypropylene, capilene, or other materials designed to wick moisture off your skin are the best ones to wear next to it. The most useful outer layer is one made of a breathable fabric such as Gore-Tex®, Versatech®, or (at a much lower cost with much the same result) one of the newer nylons. These fabrics have billions of tiny pores in them which will let moisture out but not let the wind in. A polypropylene layer next to your skin, perhaps another synthetic fabric shirt, a breathable fabric outer garment, a warm hat and gloves can make cycling or running on a bright winter's day that is not too windy very enjoyable. Generally, even when it is not windy, you will want to wear more layers when cycling than when running because of the self-generated breeze of cycling.

Shopping for Your New Sport
Internet and Mail-Order Shopping
There are very large Internet/mail-order businesses for running and cycling gear. The prices are usually lower than those found in the stores. The reputable Internet/mail-order sellers make returning items as painless as possible. I do a certain amount of mail and website ordering for some of my equipment, especially clothing. If you settle on one brand and know your proper size in it, you may also be able to buy running shoes through the Internet or mail, as I have done for years. Nevertheless, I feel that the Internet/mail-order businesses must be used with care.

You should certainly not make your first purchases through that route. For the most costly piece of equipment, the bike, you can find very attractive Iinternet/mail-ordering prices. However, your first new bike should be fitted to you, something that can be done properly only in a bike store. Furthermore, as when you buy a new car, it is a very good idea to test ride several different makes and models. Buying a bike at a distance, in my view, is not a good idea—unless you know exactly what you are looking for and have ridden it, know somebody who can put it together for you, or are confident that you can correctly assemble it yourself (Internet/mail-order bicycles come in a number of pieces) and do not care about getting after-sale service from a dealer who has an investment in you and your repeat business.

After you become somewhat knowledgeable, you can intelligently buy some of your equipment, especially clothing as noted, by mail or on the Internet. But personal advice and counsel and continuing personal service are invaluable, and you do want your local shops to stay in business. Furthermore, the Internet/mail order equipment sources cannot make adjustments to your equipment, cannot give you advice on how to use it, cannot take care of warranty repairs, and cannot be there for you in case of an equipment emergency, especially one that occurs the day before a race.

In the Stores

As a "stuff guy" myself, I have had what seems like tons of equipment during my decades-long run in the sports. Nevertheless, the most useful advice I can offer you on deciding what equipment to buy is, before doing anything, locate the best bicycle shop and the best running-shoe store in your area or, if there is one, the best du/triathlon shop. In advising you on your various choices, the staff at the better shops for both shoes and bikes (plus the needed accessories) should take into account your interests, where you are in the sport(s), what your skill levels are, and your expressed needs, as well as their own desire to make a sale. The good running shoe/bike/triathlon stores will be owned and/or staffed by athletes. The staff will have carefully evaluated the myriad number of makes and models of shoes, bikes, and equipment on the market and will have preselected a good range from which you can choose. They will make sure that the equipment fits and will stand behind their products.

I strongly suggest that you do not buy your bike in a department store or a sports super store. The prices may be very attractive, but here we are dealing with a prime case of being penny-wise and pound-foolish. Such stores generally carry only lower-end equipment, will not be equipped to handle ongoing service, and will rarely have knowledgeable sales people. At the same time, take note that not all bicycle shops are the same. Not all bike-store salespeople know what makes a good bike good and a better bike better, especially for duathlon racing. One way to judge a bicycle shop is by the most expensive bike it carries. If its cost is well above what you are going to spend, you can be reasonably confident that the staff knows what they are talking about. Also, the mechanics in the shop you patronize should be knowledgeable and willing to spend time talking with you.

Well, now that you are equipped as well as trained up, let's go racing!

CHAPTER 9

Day at the Races

This chapter is written for the first-timer, to help you get organized from the outset, and the recreational duathlete who perhaps has not been too organized, and would like to approach duathlon racing in a more organized, hopefully more productive way.

"Get Up, You Sleepy Head"

The alarm goes off at 4:30 a.m. You groggily reach over to turn it off, and just as you are about to roll over and go back to sleep you remind yourself why, at this ungodly hour, on a Saturday or Sunday of all days, you need to get out of bed. Today is the day of your first duathlon, or the first for which you have organized things properly. Hopefully you got to bed early enough last night to give yourself a reasonable number of hours of sleep. But whether you did or not, you do have to get up, now.

Let's say this is your first and let's say the race starts at 8:00 a.m. The site is an hour's drive from your home. You have decided, wisely, that for your first race it would be a good idea to get there nice and early, find a conveniently located parking place, check in before a line begins to form at the check-in desk, have plenty of time to lay out your stuff at the bike rack, attend to nature's necessities, perhaps scope out the course a bit, and even to warm up and stretch out. Actually, it's a very good idea to have this kind of schedule, whether it's your first or your 101st. I still do.

So, to get there at about 6:30 to 7:00 a.m., you need to leave the house at 5:30 to 6:00 a.m., which means, if it takes you an hour to get out of the house and load your bike and stuff on and in the car before a race (I actually allow at least seventy-five minutes for that task), getting up at 4:30–5:00 a.m. is what you'll need to do. (And yes indeed, if you are faster than I am you can get up later!) As you do so, you may well wonder, as I have done on more than one occasion, "Just why am I doing this?" Within just a few hours you will know very well why you are doing it. And if you are anything like me, you will be doing it again and again. But as you are edging out of bed for your first, second, or third race, and prodding your eyes open while standing in front of the bathroom mirror, you may well have these thoughts. Everyone does from time to time. Join the crowd.

And so it comes: apprehension, anticipation, anxiety, wonders, wondering. "Am I crazy?" "Is it too hard for me?" "Can I really do this?" occasionally interspersed with "Yes, I can really do this." And yes indeed you can. Oh what a feeling! When you started out, when you first decided to do your first race, you knew that you needed some training. You have done that. You knew that you needed to learn how to do the sport(s) you did not previously know how to do, and acquire and learn how to use the necessary equipment. You have done that, too.

For this kind of racing, you have learned that you need to do some race-specific planning and logistical preparation as well. With the help of the information in chapter 4 and this chapter, you have also done that. Now you need to set your mind on doing the race itself, you need to mentally focus all your training and your planning, your hopes and your dreams of success as you have defined it for yourself, on the race, on staying comfortable, and also on staying "within yourself." That is, you do not want to try to do anything athletically for which you are not fully prepared and capable, physically and mentally. As I have said many times in this book, like virtually all sports, duathlon is mental first, physical second. The most important thing to remember is that with your training and your planning, *if you focus, if you keep your eye on your personal goals while you are on the course*, you can do it.

First Things First

"Racing" and "doing the race." Where should your head be during your first race (or your second or third)? I'm sure you know by now that I strongly recommend that your goal for your first race (if not for every race you do, unless you are fast or have the potential to become fast) should be simply to finish, happily and healthily. That is, your first focus should be on the second of the two statements above: doing the race.

"Racing," that is, setting out to finish ahead of others in your age group, among friends, or within a different type of group (or the all-entrants group, if you are or get to be fast), can come later. As I have said before, at the beginning don't worry about speed. Just be concerned with endurance, about crossing that finish line fully in control of yourself, your senses, and your body, without a concern in the world about where you finish in relation to anyone else in the race. I have many photos of myself crossing a finish line with an expression on my face that looks like "winner," when in fact I was twentieth or fewer from last. But boy, did I have fun that day, and boy, was I proud of my finish that day.

If you like duathlon, you will surely be back for more. If you are naturally fast and/or can train up to speed, you will have plenty of opportunity to show your stuff in the future. But as you know by now, duathlon is a fairly complex sport, especially when you are new to it. Think of your first one (or even your first several) as a learning experience. And you want this first one to be fun, not a drag, not a gruelathon. So go for the finish, not for time.

Setting a Time Goal

Now, do I think that you should you never set a time goal? No, I don't. When you are ready, when you have done a few races, go ahead and do that. Make a projection of what a reasonable finish time would be for you, assuming that you will give it your best effort. Setting some reasonable time goal for yourself can add some spice to the experience. Set a goal that will take a bit of doing and some discipline in the race, but one that is realistic and reasonable. If you make it, you will feel great. If you don't (and believe me, I do not invariably meet my own projected times), there's always another race. Remember: Race performance is the product of natural ability, goal setting, training, race strategy and tactics, discipline, and the course conditions on race day. Not everything is under your control.

I will sometimes look at the time I made the previous year for a given race and set out to try to beat it. But more often than not, especially as I get older and slower, I will not look at last year's time. I don't want to pressure myself. But if I do feel like setting a time goal, often I will not set it until I'm out on the bike, experiencing how I really feel that day. Then I can make my best estimate of what I may be able to do in that race, if I put my mind to it.

Clothing and Equipment for the Race

With all the "stuff" involved in duathlon, it's very easy to forget things. Even though I've been racing for twenty-nine seasons (as of 2011), and I use a checklist of the type I present in table 9.1, I still forget things, or bring them along and then leave them back at the car or untouched in my transition-area bag. (And no, it's not age, for I have been doing the same thing for years!) But if you use a checklist, you will certainly reduce the chance that something will end up in your "forget-tery" (as my late stepmother Jeanne Erlanger Jonas liked to call it) rather than in your memory.

I will share with you here a few comments on each of the components in that checklist.

General

1. **Race directions, registration materials.** Bring along the race directions. They will be printed as part of the race application that you keep and/or will be sent to advance registrants and/or you can find them on the race's website.

Registration materials will (or should) provide you with important information, from directions to the race to a brief description of the course. For some races, a week in advance or so, you will receive a confirmation via e-mail with a link for finding your race number in advance. Having it in hand will help facilitate at-the-race check-in for you.

2. **Road and course maps.** If the race is somewhere you could not drive to in your sleep if you had to, be sure to take a road map with you. There is nothing surer to provoke prerace anxiety than getting lost on your way to it. (I know. I have done it more than once, even with a map!) If the race transition area has a street address and you have a GPS, that will help enormously in finding it! Of course, you may have also chosen to print out course maps (many races provide them on their websites), and might want to bring them along, too.

3. **USA Triathlon membership card/photo ID.** If the race is sanctioned by USA Triathlon, you will either be required to show your USAT membership card or, if you are not a member, purchase a one-day membership at the race. At many races you will also be required to show a photo ID when you check in and pick up your race packet. The transfer of a race registration to another person is strictly forbidden, for reasons of liability and fairness.

4. **Prerace clothing and shoes.** Wear whatever you are comfortable with, a warm-up suit, sweats, what have you. But do remember, even in the summertime, unless in the

middle of a heat spell, it can be cool early in the morning. It's best to be prepared, and it's always better to have too much clothing around than too little. As for shoes, it is best not to wear your running shoes to the race. Save them for the running/PaceWalking legs. I like to have a comfortable pair of moccasins or old running shoes for pre- and post-race footwear.

5. **Shoe horn.** Very helpful for getting into both bike and run shoes quickly. This, however, is one item that I frequently forget to use.

6. **Digital watch.** If you don't want to keep track of your own race time(s), this is obviously one you don't need. But if you're compulsive like some of us you may want a watch that records and saves split times (that is, your times for each segment of the race, including the transitions), marking off individual leg and transition times, and for a personal record. However, since most races now give you a digital timing chip to put around your ankle before the start, your split times will be recorded with your overall time and appear on the race website with the final race results.

7. **Magic marker.** Only in my thirteenth season or so did it occur to me that I could skip the prerace line that always seems to go on forever (no matter how short it is). That's the one to have a race volunteer put your race number on your arms and legs with magic marker, required at almost every race for easy competitor ID by the race-timers. If you have your own marker, you need only note where the

number is to be placed and have it put there either by a friend or loved one who is with you (before you enter the transition area, where visitors are not allowed) or by a fellow racer at the bike rack.

8. **Glasses, sunglasses.** If you wear prescription glasses, and in the race plan to use prescription sunglasses or bike goggles with a prescription insert as I do, I think that it's still a good idea to bring along your regular glasses as well as your sunglasses or goggles. Then you have a backup. Of course, if you start out for the race before the sun is fully up, you will have your regular glasses with you in any case.

9. **Extra safety pins.** At the race check-in there will almost invariably be a supply of safety pins available, to be used for attaching your race numbers to your clothing, as required. If you do get into the sport you may want to buy a "race number belt," an elastic strap with attachment points for your running race number that goes around your waist. Nevertheless, for backup, I always have a few safety pins in my kit.

10. **Towel(s).** Bring at least one towel to dry off a bit after the first sweaty run and to dry off with at the end of the race.

11. **Keys/money pouch.** I always carry my car keys on me, either in a little pouch clipped on the waist of my liner shorts, at the small of my back, or, if I am wearing a bike jersey for the whole race (which I often do) in one of those three pockets you find at the back. When I am alone at a race, in the same spot I also carry a sports wallet with a

credit card and some cash (as well as the usually required photo ID and, if it's a USAT sanctioned race, my USAT card).

12. **Food.** You may want to have a little something just before the race, either real food or an energy bar or gel (see also below, on prerace eating). While at most races food, from bagels and fruit on up, is supplied at the end, hey, you never know.

13. **Fresh clothing for after the race.** This can be the same as your prerace clothing or, if you expect it to be a hot day, it might simply be a clean T-shirt and a pair of shorts. If you have worn nonrunning shoes to the race, you will be very happy to be able to step into them at the appropriate time.

14. **Sunscreen.** Useful both before and after the race, if there is a bright sun out.

15. **Ground cover/plastic garbage bag.** I always bring an old bathmat to use as a ground cover on which to lay out my race stuff. If the ground might be damp, it is very useful to have a plastic garbage bag to put under it.

Runs/PaceWalks

16. **Singlet/T-shirt/bike shirt, shorts, socks.** There are choices to be made here. I always wear a bike jersey for the whole race. If you've got one, that's what I suggest doing. Otherwise, unless it is chilly, you might want to wear a racing singlet for the run, then put a T-shirt over it for the

bike (which can get breezy), and then doff it for the second run. Also, please note that for USAT sanctioned races, you must wear a shirt/top at all times during the race. Whatever shorts you are going to wear for the bike, you should also wear for the runs. I wear bike socks, as you know. Either bike socks or running socks of the proper type (not too heavy) will work for both the bike and the run. Or, if you've got running and bike shoes that fit really well so that you won't get blisters, you may decide to do both without socks,

17. **Cap, sweat-band.** I find a cap very helpful for cooling when running or PaceWalking in the direct sunlight, while also wearing a sweatband. I may take the cap off when I'm in the shade, usually alternating it with the sweatband. Also available are caps with built-in sweatbands, a very nice (but not especially inexpensive) alternative.

18. **Running shoes.** Again, like the bike, you don't want to forget them. While you can bike in your running shoes with the proper pedals, you know by now that there is no way you can run in your bike shoes.

19. **Wind-shell, long-sleeve T-shirt, tights.** If you do early or late season races in cold weather, you may well want to have some extra protection, perhaps even a balaclava for your head and face on the bike if it's really cold and windy. Sometimes in early and late season races when it is brisk but not too cold, I'll wear a pair of tights on the first run and the bike and then peel them off quickly in the second transition, for the second run, after I am all nice and warmed up.

On the Bike

20. **Bicycle.** Has anyone ever arrived at a duathlon without their bike? Yes. Rarely, to be sure, but yes. That's why it's on the Checklist.

21. **Bicycle front wheel.** Has anyone ever arrived at a duathlon with their bike but without the front wheel for it? Yes. Rarely, to be sure, but yes. If you are driving to a race and putting your bike in the car, most often you will take the front wheel off to do so. Also, with many car-top bike racks like the one that I use, you will do the same thing. Actually, I did end up volunteering at one of Dan Honig's Harriman State Park (New York) triathlons a while back when I arrived with my bike but no front wheel. I was much too far from home to go back to get the wheel that was, thankfully, still sitting in my carport when I returned from the race. That's why it's now on the Checklist as a separate item.

22. **Bicycle pump, full-size.** Once again, if you are cycling to the race from home, of course you will want to top up your tires before you go out the door. If you are driving, top up at the car in the parking lot so that you don't have to carry your pump to the transition area and have extra clutter at your space.

23. **Bicycle pump, frame-fit/CO$_2$ cartridge.** It is difficult to get racing tires pumped up to the correct pressure with a frame-fit pump. But you must have one with you on the road for that emergency you hope will never come. I carry

a pump even when I bring a CO_2 cartridge or an inflator-with-goo along. You never know if the latter is going to work right or if, heaven forebid, you get two flats.

24. **Water bottles.** As I have noted, I use one twenty-ounce water bottle filled with my favorite energy drink for the bike leg in a sprint-distance duathlon, unless it is an extra-long bike leg (and on occasion they can be up to 20 miles, for which I will carry two). You may also want to have an extra at the transition area so that you can drink easily during the transitions.

25. **Bike seat bag w/spare tube and tools.** The bag should be as small and light as possible while still accommodating the essentials.

26. **Computer.** Make sure to put in a fresh battery at the beginning of the season. It's not fun to have your computer go blank just at the beginning of the bike leg, as happened to me once in an ironman distance triathlon.

27. **Bike shoes, gloves, helmet.** If you forget your bike shoes, you can always ride wearing your running shoes, but if you are used to wearing bike shoes, you will want to have them with you. Also while you can use running shoes on clipless pedals, that is not fun. The platform is very small and your foot will be slipping off constantly. Bike gloves make for comfort but are certainly not essential (and those competitors going for speed don't usually spend the time necessary to put them on—though I do). However,

as you surely know by now, you will not be allowed to do the race without a helmet. Therefore you need to have it with you. At many races there is at least one plaintive announcement made before the start asking if anyone has an extra helmet they could loan to a forgetful person. Now you don't want to be in that position, do you?

28. **Bike shirt, shorts, liner shorts, socks.** Again, as you know by now, for comfort I wear liner shorts under my bike shorts, I wear my bike outfit for the whole duathlon, and I wear socks for both the runs and the bike. With experience, you will be making your own choices for the various combinations.

29. **Jacket, long-sleeve shirt, tights.** It is unlikely that you will be racing in cold weather early in your career, but, hey, you never know.

30. **Tissues.** A very helpful item for such things as cleaning the sweat off glasses during a long bike ride. I always have it on my list. But then again I almost invariably forget to stick them into the bike jersey pocket where it would be so nice to have them.

Race Day Preparation and Check-In
Eating and Drinking before the Race
Everyone has an eating program to recommend, and the recommendations vary widely. I've tried a variety of approaches over the years. As you certainly know by now, I go relatively

Table 9.1
The Pre-Race Checklist
GENERAL
Race directions, registration materials
Road maps
GENERAL
USA Triathlon membership card/photo ID
Pre-race clothing, warm-up suit/sweats
Shoe horn
Digital watch
Magic Marker
Glasses, sun-glasses
Extra safety pins
Keys/money pouch
Towel(s)
Food
Fresh clothing for after the race
Sunscreen
Ground cover/plastic garbage bag
RUNS/PACEWALKS
Singlet/T-shirt, shorts, socks
Cap, sweat-band
Running shoes
Wind-shell, long-sleeve T-shirt, tights
BIKE
Bicycle
Bicycle front wheel

Bicycle pump, full-size
Bicycle pump, frame-fit
Water bottle(s)
Seat bag w/spare tube and tools
Computer
Bike shoes, gloves, helmet
BIKE
Bike shirt, shorts, liner shorts, socks
Jacket, long-sleeve shirt, tights
Tissues

slowly in the races. Therefore, I am likely to be burning primarily fat stores for energy. I have found that since that is the case, it doesn't matter too much what I eat the night before, as long as it doesn't leave me feeling overfull and uncomfortable or lead to bowel problems, which can a be nuisance on race day. On the other hand, if you go even moderately fast, carbohydrates are important, and you should consider carbohydrate loading. You can certainly consult one of the performance-oriented tri/duathlon publications for advice on that subject (see chapter 12). However, it is most likely that you will use the trial-and-error method over time to arrive at what works best for you. This is exactly what I have done over the years, and still do as I modify this or that routine.

However, for everyone, prerace hydration is very important. Start drinking fluids several days before the race to get hydrated, especially if it is likely to be hot. At the same time, try not to overdo it—then you will not have to spend excess time spilling the excess before and/or during the race. Again, trial and error is the long-run method to determine just what works best for *you*.

As to eating on the morning of the race, there are as many approaches to it as there are to eating in the days just before it. You want to eat something, perhaps a piece of fruit and a roll or a sweet bun, a bit of cheese, an energy bar or two, with fluids. Although other authorities disagree, I suggest staying away from coffee. Caffeine, of course, helps to wake you up and increase your level of alertness. However, it also stimulates the kidneys. Too much kidney activity can become a real nuisance before and during a race. As for eating, the important thing is not to overeat, not to give yourself a full, uncomfortable feeling that can be especially bothersome on the first run.

The Night Before
The night before the race, it is a good idea to have every-thing that you will be wearing in the morning set out, and to have the bag(s)/backpack with the rest of the stuff that you will taking packed and ready to go. Most folks will try to have one backpack or sports equipment bag with all the stuff, to make it convenient to carry from the parking area to check-in and the transition area. When you subsequently lay out your equipment next to your bike in the transition area, you will naturally separate it into little sport-specific piles, but you don't necessarily have to do that in your race bag/pack.

Arrival

When you arrive at the parking area, unload your bike carefully. No reason to damage it at this point! If you have removed the front tire, reinstall it, make sure to reset the release lever on the front brake (if you don't know what I am referring to here, have your bike person show it to you when in the shop sometime), and make sure the wheel is spinning freely. If one side is rubbing on a brake pad, release the brake again and then make sure that the wheel mounts are centered properly between the prongs of the fork. As previously noted, it is a good idea to pump up your bicycle tires at the car. If you have not previously set your bike in a lower gear so that you can get started comfortably on the bike leg, do it here.

Racking Your Bike

If you know your race number (see Race Directions, No. 1, above), you can first go to the transition area and rack your bike. The transition area is a flat, open space, usually either a paved section of a parking lot or a grassy area, convenient to the race start/finish. As you know by now, it is here that provision is made for keeping your bike and your other racing stuff. At most races, you will find the racks numbered. You must use the correct one or risk disqualification. There is an occasional race that uses a "rack wherever you want to" system. In that case, it is important to note some landmark or bearing so that you can easily find the rack when you are coming back to it after the first run. There are two modes for bike-racking: with the brake handles draped over the bar or with the seat tongue on it. Unless you are first, follow the dictum, when in Rome, do what the Romans do. If you are first to your rack, ask a volunteer which way your bike should be mounted.

Try not to arrive at the last minute, even if you have done many races. Your assigned bike rack will then be crowded and you will have to take whatever space and location on it are left. Last-minute arrival also increases your chances of forgetting something important along the way. Either way, once your bike is racked, you will lay out your run and bike stuff on the ground on one side of your bike.

Checking In

With or without your bike in hand, proceed to the check-in desk(s). Of course, for races that have day-of-the-race registration, if you have not preregistered you will go to the registration line. The more popular races generally do not have day-of-the-race registration. In any case, I strongly recommend preregistration. You will avoid what can be a frustrating, anxiety-provoking experience enduring what can seem to be an interminable wait in a long, slow-moving line. (I must say that being somewhat compulsive in certain [ahem!] areas, on this one I speak not from experience, but only from observation.) Extra, unnecessary anxiety is something you just don't need. Check-in for prerace registrants usually proceeds quite quickly. You will be given a plastic bag or manila envelope called the race packet, and at races that provide souvenir T-shirts (most of them now do), that item as well. You will then most likely be directed to a separate table where you will pick up your timing chip, assigned by your race number. Once you have your race packet and timing chip in hand, proceed back to the transition area.

In the Transition Area: Before the Start

In the race packet you will find at a minimum the race numbers to attach to your race shirt and your bike. There may also be a sticker with your number to be attached to your bike helmet. You may in addition find assorted goodies, ranging from a sports nutrition bar, to a copy of one of the triathlon publications, to a race souvenir, plus announcements of upcoming races run by the same race director/organization. Whereas there are still occasional races where you will receive separate shirt numbers for the runs and the bike, most assume that you will be wearing the same shirt for the runs and the bike and thus provide a single number. It will usually have a tear-off tab at the bottom to be collected by the timers at the finish. If you are using safety pins, put it on the front of your race-shirt, because at the finish your number must be on your front. If you have a race belt, you can wear the number on the front for the first run, slide it around to your back (out of the way and the breeze) for the bike, and slide it back around to the front for the second run. As for the timing chip, you will wrap the Velcro® strip to which it is attached around one ankle.

There will also usually be a number for your bike printed on an adhesive-backed paper, or one that has two adhesive strips, either one to be folded over the bike's top-tube, or seat tube (the piece that connects the handlebar stem to the vertical tube on which the seat is mounted), with the two sides stuck together. You may also find that you have enough room to mount it on the seat tube itself, or one of the rear chain stays. In either of those locations, it is out of the way. At your transition area spot, arrange your bike stuff in some order that makes sense to you. Although you don't have to be compulsive about it, develop something of a prerace routine, and don't be tempted to change it. On the few occasions when I have strayed far afield, I have not ended up a happy camper.

Warm-up

The walking back and forth, car to transition area to check-in, will help you limber up and warm up some. I usually do a bit of an organized warm-up before a duathlon. You can jog a bit, for two to ten minutes. You can stretch a bit. But don't try any stretches that are not part of your regular routine. You can end up pulling a muscle once you get out on the run. You can possibly bike a bit, although few people do that. But you certainly can, and after a few races you will know if you need to do so. The amount of warming up you do will be partially determined by how much extra time you have available. That in turn will be determined by such factors as when you arrived at the race, how long check-in took, whether you have to use the toilet or not, and if so, how long the line was. If the race is starting later in the morning than duathlons usually do (7:30 to 8:00 a.m.), do remember to stay out of the sun.

Getting to the Start

Usually about fifteen minutes or so before the start, the race director will make a series of announcements. It is a good idea to listen to them, even if you have done that particular race before. He or she will describe the course, talk about safety issues, and of most immediate importance to you at this point, describe the transition area exits and entrances for the first run and the bike. If you don't know where to come in from the first run, go out on the bike, come in from the bike, and go out on the second run, you can waste a lot of time during the race finding out. Of course there will almost always be volunteers to point you in the right direction(s), but it is good to have the information in your head just the same.

At the end of the announcements, you will be directed to the starting line. Seed yourself according to your expected speed on the first run. If you are an eight-minutes-per-mile person, you can be in the middle of the pack. If you are a ten-minutes-per-mile or slower person (like me) I suggest getting toward the back. Actually, I always start from the rear, and as I get older and even slower, remain there. But it is much more fun to start too far back in the pack and pass people as you get into your rhythm than it is to start too far forward and have people virtually running over you for the first few hundred yards.

And finally, then, the horn goes off and you are racing!

The First Run
The first rule of the first run is, "Don't go out too fast." The second and third rules are exactly the same. Especially in your first race, or one still early in your racing career, you will have little if any idea of just how fast you can go in the first run and still have plenty left for the bike and the second run.

So do play it safe. You will know from your training what is a comfortable pace for you. The adrenalin will be flowing, for sure. But just try to stay within yourself, which means doing what you know your body can do, in the context of the training you have done. If you do feel like "turning it on," I suggest saving that for the second run or at least for the bike.

First Run-Bike Transition

Once again, make sure that you know where your bike is so you can head directly for it once you re-enter the transition area. If it's a hot day and you have worked up a sweat, you may want to towel off a bit, but don't worry about getting completely dry. You will dry off completely soon enough in the breeze of the bike ride, and then will you start sweating again soon enough after that. Try to remember to drink some water, juice, or energy drink while you are putting on your bike shoes (if you are changing shoes), sunglasses, helmet, and (if you are like me) gloves. Head for the bike exit, either walking or trotting, and mount up where you are told to, not sooner. Do not attempt to ride through the transition area. That will almost certainly get you disqualified, but more importantly, it could get you or someone else injured.

If you want to keep your transition time down, you will need to plan it out. You could even practice your transitions. I don't do this, and it shows in my high transition times. They drive my wife crazy, but they help to relax me, and my overall race performance, in terms of comfort as well as time, may benefit from the extra couple of minutes of relative rest. However, if working up to fast transitions is something that is or will become important to you, you may want to work on transitioning.

The Bike

The bike ride is fairly straightforward. In the races you will be doing (that is, unless you have worked your way up to the elite-racer category, in which case you will hardly be looking at this book!) drafting on riders in front of you is not permitted. (Drafting on is riding in the slipstream of a rider in front of you so as to shield yourself from the aerodynamic drag that other riders are experiencing.) This is not Tour de France–style peloton racing. You are essentially doing a time trial (racing against the clock) with a large group of other riders doing the same thing. As with the first run, my suggestion is not to go out too fast, even though you may be very excited to have finished that first run. Don't worry about passing or being passed. Get comfortable. Get into your own zone. Ride your own race.

Remember to use your water bottles with whatever liquid you have chosen to have in them. That's what they are there for. If you wait to drink until you are feeling dry, you have waited too long and will not be able to catch up at any point during the race. That's simply the way our bodies work. There are a variety of sports drinks on the market, as you know. Trial and error will tell you which one of them will work better for you (and some folks like just plain water).

If you have had a chance to go over the bike course before the race, either on your bike or in a car, you will know where the significant hills, if any, are. Make sure that you get down into a low enough gear to make any hill comfortably, before you start up it. You don't want to kill your legs going up a hill, and it can be tough downshifting while going up a fairly steep one. As the same time, take it easy on the downhills. The last thing you want to do is spin out and crash. I find that I am comfortable up to about 35 miles per hour on a long downhill. (Fast riders may get up to 60!) Anything over that and I will start braking a bit. Staying upright on the bike is a nice feeling. Going over isn't.

When you get to the last mile or two of the bike, start taking it a bit easy. Don't hammer all the way in. Drop your gear down a notch or two lower than you would usually set it for that terrain so that you can pedal easily. You will likely be finding out soon enough about the difficulties many duathletes have in making the bike-to-run changeover, at least when they are first starting out racing. Many find that spinning at a higher cadence than their usual one for the last quarter to half mile is very helpful.

Bike-Second Run Transition

Dismount where you are told to. Make sure you know where your place on the bike racks was before you left, so that you won't have to waste time wandering around the transition area looking for your pile of stuff. You will doff your helmet, take off your gloves if you wore them, and put your running shoes back on if you rode in bike shoes. Take a drink while you are changing up, either from a water bottle you have set aside for that purpose, or from one still on the bike with fluid in it. Walk or at most jog gently through the transition area to the exit for the second run. If you are anything like most of the rest of us, you will find your legs feeling somewhat funny under you. That's why, by the way, it's a good idea to do two to three "bricks" (bike-run workouts) during your training. You will have some idea of what is coming.

The Second Run

The main thing about the second run is getting started. Finishing it (and the race!) will take care of itself. But your legs may well feel funny. For a sprint-distance duathlon, you will have just come off of thirty to sixty minutes (or perhaps more) of heavy use of your front thigh muscles (the quadriceps or quads) for biking, and you are asking your legs to immediately convert to primarily using the muscles at the back of your thighs (the hamstrings) and your calf muscles for running. Your hamstrings have been sitting there passively for the most part, and the blood flow in your legs has been going primarily to your quads.

So you need to loosen up your hamstrings and get the blood flowing to them. That usually takes some time. Sometimes it takes me up to a mile before I feel comfortable running or even doing the PaceWalking race gait. In a sprint-distance duathlon, that means that I am just getting loose as I cross the finish line! But sometimes I get loose in less than a mile, and that may be your experience, too. Just go with the flow, don't try to push it, and you will be all right. If you are tired or tight during the second run and need to ordinary walk for a time, that's fine. Don't worry about it. Many people have done it. Remember. The important thing is finishing, and walking is perfectly legal in a duathlon.

The Finish

And that brings us to the finish. Oh what a feeling when you finish your first! (As you know by now, for me the feeling has been there in almost every one of the 220-plus duathlons and triathlons that I have done.) Remember to remember that very first finish, to savor it, to value it. You will finish your first duathlon only once in your life. If you have liked the experience of training and racing, you will surely do it again, and again. But that very first one marks a special time, a special place for you, regardless of where you finish in relation to everyone else in the race.

Smile, laugh, shout, jump up and down, dance a celebratory jig, raise both arms above your head in triumph, even have a bit of a cry (and I have done that more than once, I can tell you), regardless of your finishing time. For, you have done something very special for yourself, especially if you have not come from a racing or athletic background (and numerous recreational duathletes, like myself, have not), something that not too many other people in the world have done. Yes, it is a time to remember, proudly.

Three Final Questions

First, do you need to go through all the stuff I have written about in this chapter each time you race? I can tell you that you almost never will. I find it hard to remember everything I've written down here. You probably will, too. Each time, I do try to make sure to do the stuff that I regard as most important, particularly for the safety items, and to be certain that I have with me all the essentials for registration and racing. As for the rest, I do *try* to remember. Some days I am more successful at it than others. So I would suggest that you, too, should try to pick out what's important for you and try to do those things each time.

Second, and much more importantly, will you have a good time each time you race? Well, as long as you train properly and choose your races so that they will be suitable for you, you almost always will.

Third, will you always enjoy the finish? Again, unless it's a totally dreadful day weatherwise, too hot and humid, too cold and windy, damp, even rainy (I generally don't race in the rain, even though years ago I did that first biathlon in the rain) or you are undertrained, or have chosen an unsuitable race, yes, you almost always will.

And now that you have finished your Day at the Races, you are ready for your Night at the Opera.*

---

* For the younger set reading this book (and almost all of you will be younger than me) a three-man group called the Marx Brothers were among the most famous American comedians of the 1930s and 40s. Their two most famous movies were, you guessed it, *A Day at the Races* and *A Night at the Opera*.

CHAPTER 10

Duathlon as Part of a Total Program for Healthy Living

There are duathletes who go fast, and as I have said on more than one occasion in this book, more power to them. But for me one of the best things about duathlon, and the other forms of multisport racing, is that, as I have also said on more than one occasion in this book, the duathlon is for everyone, fast, slow, and in between. For many of us who do it, fast, slow, or in between, it's just plain fun, and that's why we do it. It's also a great way to get in shape and stay in shape. Duathlon can even become for you the center of living a healthy lifestyle, beyond just staying in shape. In this chapter we are going to look at how becoming and being a duathlete can do that for you.

The Basic Ten of Health

Defining *what* healthy living is, is not complicated. *Living* a healthy lifestyle can be. It takes thought, organization, and planning. It then takes careful, consistent, and ongoing implementation. The key is that you really have to want to do it. As the old joke goes, "How many psychiatrists does it take to change a light bulb? Just one. But the light bulb really has to want to change."

These are a Basic Ten of activities and behaviors that are central to healthy living.

1. Exercising regularly

2. Managing one's weight

3. Eating a healthy diet

4. Not using tobacco products, or prescription psychoactive drugs on a nonprescription basis

5. Safely using other nonprescription mood-altering drugs, including ethyl alcohol

6. Managing one's internal and external stressors effectively

7. Using safe sexual practices

8. Protecting personal safety in and out of the home, including in the automobile and at the workplace.

9. Maintaining one's immune status at an effective level

10. Undergoing periodic health and wellness appraisals.

Duathlon Training and Racing as Part of an Overall Personal Health Promotion Program
Taking Time Indefinitely

To a greater or lesser extent, as we've learned, undertaking each of the Basic Ten involves mobilizing your motivation.

Some of the listed items are harder to do than others. But the process of motivation mobilization works for all the personal health-promoting behaviors listed above. Mobilizing your motivation to become and be a regular exerciser is particularly useful for setting you up to move ahead in one or more of the other elements of the Basic Ten. Why? Because there is only one other health-promoting activity on the list that takes time that you were previously spending on doing other things, on an ongoing basis. (That one is being a recovering alcoholic/substance abuser and going to group for an indefinite period of time.)

Exercising regularly takes time especially dedicated to it, for as long as you do it. For all of the others (with the noted exception), if there is any commitment of extra time, it is limited. For example, let's say you go to an organized weight-loss program to learn how to eat in a healthy manner. It lasts for a finite period of time. Once you have learned how to do that, and incorporate what you have learned into your pattern of daily living, you will find that food shopping, cooking, and eating take just about the same amount of time, whether you are doing it in a healthy or an unhealthy manner.

So, remembering that the hard part of regular exercise is the regular, not the exercise, if you can become a regular exerciser you will have shown yourself that you really can take charge of your life in a significant way. You have been able to say to yourself, "I am willing to spend time doing something that is both fun and good for my health (and on those days when it might not be so much fun, doing it anyway), rather than spending that time doing something else."

Cross-training and Its Advantages

By training for duathlon racing you are engaging in cross training. Cross training is working out in two or more sports as part of the same training program, and it is even healthier than single-sport training. First, in the two duathlon sports, you are using two different major muscle groups, thereby increasing your strength and endurance for both at the same time. Second, by doing less of each sport as part of your overall training program, you are reducing the risk of overuse injury in either one. Third, you are reducing the risk of boredom that for some can accompany doing just one sport.

The 2008 Physical Activity Guidelines for Americans

In 2008, the US Department of Health and Human Services published the then most-recent *Physical Activity Guidelines for Americans* (www.health.gov/paguidelines). The guidelines recommend that to promote a basic level of health, adults should do 150 minutes per week of moderate exercise, with a higher level of benefit to be derived from doing up to 300 minutes a week of vigorous exercise. The sprint-distance duathlon training program would place you right in the middle of the USDHHS recommendations for achieving and maintaining a healthy level of physical fitness, over a thirteen-week period. What a great way to meet these recommendations, don't you think?

Racing to Train and Training to Race

In considering the relationship between racing and training for the distance sports like running, cycling, and swimming, folks who do them generally fall into two groups. There are those like me who, first, enjoy the racing for the pure fun of it. But second, we race to train in the sense that we wouldn't train as much as we do if we were not racing. At any rate, I am quite sure that I for one would not have been training the way I have been for more than three decades were I not racing. Then, there are the folks, usually the faster ones among us, who are training to race. They have certain time and distance goals that they want to achieve in the races and in order to achieve them they need to engage in certain amounts and types of training that will go well beyond the USDHHS minimums.

Either one is fine. Either one can be fun. Racing to train almost always is. Training to race certainly can be. But it can become not so much fun over time. That's where proper goal setting (discussed in chapter 3) comes in. First, given your genetic endowment and natural abilities (or lack thereof) and those of your potential competitors, you need to set realistic racing goals in terms of results, speeds, and distances; otherwise, you won't achieve your goals, which could very easily lead to frustration and even anger. Second, if you're not careful, you may find yourself overtraining in order to achieve certain race results that on paper look realistic but in fact may not be. This can lead to unnecessary pain, to injury, to the de-emphasizing of other important parts of your life, like family and performing well at work. It may lead, eventually, to quitting. This is definitely not to say that if you have the ability and the potential to go fast and win, overall or in your age group, you shouldn't go for it. Of course, you should. It is to say that in order to make racing and training part of your overall healthy lifestyle, balance has to be achieved too (see Step 4 of the Ordinary Mortals® Pathway to Mobilizing Motivation, below).

The Ordinary Mortals® Pathway to Mobilizing Motivation

As you already know, regular exercise is one of the Basic Ten of health. Becoming a regular exerciser by becoming a duathlete can have a special role to play in helping you to adopt a healthy lifestyle, if you are not there already. For me, how you go about mobilizing and maintaining your motivation to do so is at the center of engaging in any personal health-promoting behavior. You want to be able to mobilize it effectively. We discussed the Ordinary Mortals® Pathway to Mobilizing Motivation in a bit of detail in chapter 3. Here we will go over it in more detail.

I developed the Ordinary Mortals® Pathway over time from observation, anecdotal interviews, and experience. While it has not been tested experimentally, it appears to be a logical approach to crossing the bridge from thinking about and planning for, to actively engaging in one or more of the behaviors that constitute healthy living. Further, it is one of the two accepted pathways to mobilizing motivation that appear in the *American College of Sports Medicine's Exercise is Medicine,* the textbook for that ACSM program that I was privileged to co-author (with Dr. Edward Phillips) and from which parts of this chapter are drawn. It happens to be a health-promoting "medication" that appears to have no potential negative side effects.

Motivation Is All in Your Mind

Motivation is a thought or set of thoughts, not something tangible. And except in self-destructive people, motivation is always there in one's mind, for it is essential to self-preservation and the underlying human striving to be healthy. "Getting motivated" is not a question of developing or importing the mind state. It is not finding the magic outside of yourself and somehow bringing it inside. It is, rather, a matter of activating a potential mental activity that is presently quiescent, of locating it inside yourself, of removing roadblocks you yourself may have placed in the way of its expression, and then as we say, mobilizing it, getting it going, getting it working for you. Indeed, at its most basic level, *motivation is a mental process that links a thought or a feeling with an action.*

The Phases of the Pathway

There are three phases in the process of finding or developing motivation. The first, is having emotional and/or intellectual thoughts that are potentially motivating. The second is establishing a clear mental pathway between those thoughts and the potential for taking the related action. The third is taking the action as the result of phases one and two. As discussed briefly in chapter 3, The Ordinary Mortals® Pathway has five steps:

1. Assessment, both self and, if indicated, professional.

2. Defining success for yourself. To be effective success has to be defined within your own context, it has to be realistic for you, and achievement of it has to be reasonably within the realm of possibility for you.

3. Goal setting. As you know by now, this is the central element of the Ordinary Mortals® Pathway.

4. Establishing priorities among the various sectors of your life and between the several goals you have set for yourself. This is particularly important for achieving success as you become a duathlete.

5. Taking control of the whole process. This final step itself has six elements of its own (see below).

While you go through this process, it will be very helpful for you if make some notes, write some things down. *Writing down thoughts definitely focuses the mind.*

Step 1. Assessment

Assessment has two components, assessment by oneself and assessment by others, usually health professionals. As we shall see, self-assessment is closely connected to goal setting. In self-assessment, the focus is asking yourself questions like, Where am I now in my life? How did I get here? What do I like about myself, my body? What do I not like? What is it about my body and mind that I am unhappy with, that could be positively affected by exercising regularly and beyond that, Doin' the Du? What would I like to change, if anything, and why? Where am I now in my physical-activity level? Have I tried regular exercise before and failed to stick with it? At the present time, what do I estimate my potential to stick with an exercise program to be? Realism is very important here.

What unmet personal needs am I thinking about attempting to meet? Am I ready, really ready, to try it? Would I really like to change, even if it means giving up something I am accustomed to? Do I think I can mobilize the mental strength (and it does take mental strength—there are no magic bullets to significantly change a personal behavior) if that is what I want or need to do? What has my previous experience been with personal health behavior change? Good? Bad? Some success? None? What can I learn from that experience for this time?

Then there is the matter of professional assessment. This is not a medical book, and the following is not to be taken as medical advice. Most otherwise healthy folks do not have to seek medical advice before engaging in regular exercise. However, it would be a very good idea to consult your physician before starting out if you have one or more of the following diseases or conditions: previous heart attack; chest pain, pressure, or severe shortness of breath on exertion; lung disease, especially chronic obstructive pulmonary disease; and/or bone, joint or other musculoskeletal diseases or other limitations. You also might want to consult your physician, just to be on the safe side, if you have any of the following: high blood pressure, high blood cholesterol, diabetes or any other chronic illness, or if you use one or more prescription medications on a regular basis, abuse drugs or alcohol, smoke, have a family history of heart disease, or are overweight by twenty pounds or more.

Step 2. Defining Success for Oneself
How you approach the subject of success can be either very helpful or rather harmful in the process of setting and

achieving goals. Whether it concerns becoming a regular exerciser, how to stop smoking, or losing weight, just how you define success for yourself will have a major impact on the outcome. To be helpful and facilitating for health-promoting behavior change, success must be defined in terms that make sense for you and must be realistically achievable. If success is defined in terms that are either objectively impossible or very difficult to achieve, then striving to achieve it becomes frustrating, inhibiting, anger provoking and will eventually lead to quitting.

For example, if you are naturally slow afoot and decide to take up running as part of becoming a duathlete, you shouldn't define success in terms of absolute speed, for example by saying to yourself, "I will consider myself successful when I can run a mile in eight minutes." Success, in your case, might be better defined in terms of endurance, so a better statement for you might be, "As my first objective, I want to be able to run for twenty minutes without stopping, at a comfortable pace." Once that objective is achieved, another can be set, if you want to do so. For success must also be defined with the recognition that its meaning for you can change over time. In fact, for most people who experience success in regular exercise, it will change over time. However, at the beginning of the process, there is no way of knowing just how far any one individual will get.

Finally, you must consider "endowment" (genetic potential) and "enhancement" (what you can do with it). Whatever the proportion is between endowment and enhancement as the factors determining the achievement of success, very few people have the genetic potential for developing the body of a world-class body builder (even if they were to use steroids), and very few have the potential of looking like a glamorous movie star (even with the assistance of plastic surgery). Nor do many people have it physically within themselves to run a marathon in under three hours. In setting your goals for exercise, it is important to recognize the role your genetic makeup plays in determining what you can potentially do (or not do). Which leads us to goal setting.

Step 3. Goal Setting

Goal setting is the central element of the pathway. What is it that I want to do, and why do I want to do it? Where do I want to get? Why do I want to get there? For whom would I be making the change—others, or myself, or both? What do I expect to get out of the change should I achieve it? What do I think I can reasonably expect to accomplish? Do I want to reduce my future risk for acquiring various diseases and negative health conditions? What do I hope to feel and be when I have made the contemplated changes in my life? Very importantly, what are the "give-ups," and can I, do I want to, commit to them? Arriving at satisfactory answers to these questions for oneself is absolutely key. Doing so provides the focus and the concentration one must have in order to have the best chance of success in the chosen endeavor.

The initial goals you set must be reasonable ones at the time you set them. Recognizing that what is considered to be realistic is likely to change over time, nothing can kill a change process faster than the setting of unrealistic, unachievable goals. Once you have established your goals, everything else, from planning a workout schedule to buying a pair of running shoes or a bicycle, to implementing the plan on a regular basis, then follows along with an inherent logic that relates to your goals, ones designed to work for you. The establishment of goals creates the mindset, the mental environment, which will permit and then facilitate what for most people is a major change in the way they live. It is the thinking that gets you going and keeps you going on an organized way, right up to the starting of your first, or your next, duathlon.

Step 4. Establishing Priorities

Establishing priorities for your planned duathlon training program and the balance of your life is the next step. Creating balance is central to making the whole process work. If you have set more than one goal, how do you rank them? Then, what about priorities between the new goal(s) and other important parts of your life, like relationships with family and friends, and employment? If juggling needs to be done, it will be helpful to do some thinking about that and yes, set priorities.

As I have noted on more than one occasion, becoming a regular exerciser takes time for the rest of your life. Thus finding the time and making the time is central to achieving success. This aspect of the enterprise should not be swept under the rug. It needs to be examined carefully. How is your time being spent now? Can you give up four to five hours of television a week? Can you get up forty-five minutes earlier four to five days a week (including the two weekend days) and cut down on dawdling time by fifteen minutes on each of those days? Can your spouse, for example, do some of the food shopping and cooking and help with some household chores? It will be very helpful to think about these matters as part of your overall planning process.

Step 5. *Taking Control*

This is the final step. Taking Control itself has six elements to it, to help you get to where the Ordinary Mortals® Pathway to Mobilizing Motivation is intended to lead you. That taking control of your life means running your life instead of letting it run you is self-explanatory but a difficult challenge for many of us to meet. Taking control, for yourself" is critical to locating, unblocking, and then mobilizing motivation. When you take control, you have decided what you want to do with your body, perhaps to do something you have never done, or even contemplated doing, before. Like doing your first duathlon.

We have already considered the first two elements in some detail. Let us look at the others, briefly. No. 3, Dealing with the fear of failure, means just what it says. Giving yourself permission to fail can be, for many, marvelously liberating and actually help you significantly in navigating the pathway to success. There are many reasons for failure in becoming a regular exerciser; none of them have moral content. You are not a bad person if you don't make it this time around. You can always try again, and if you never make it, well you just don't and that should be the end of it.

No. 4, Exploring your limits while recognizing your limitations, means injecting realism into your program, as we have noted. Play to your strengths, but at the same time deal with your weaknesses realistically. Once having embarked on the journey of regular exercise and becoming and being a

---

The Six Keys to Taking Control

1. Understanding that motivation is not a thing, but a process that links a thought or feeling with an action.

2. Following the first four steps of the Ordinary Mortals® Pathway to Mobilizing Your Motivation, from the beginning.

3. Dealing with the fear of failure.

4. Being ready to explore your limits while recognizing your limitations.

5. Understanding that it is gradual change that leads to permanent changes.

6. Understanding that we can never be perfect; we can always get better.

---

duathlete, you may take your mind and your body to places you never dreamed of. I knew from the get-go, in both duathlon and triathlon, that I was never going to be fast. That was my limitation. But by my third season in multisport racing, I began exploring my limits as to distance. And yes, I completed my first half-ironman distance triathlon and then my first ironman that year. I did my first long duathlon the next year. Does this mean that you have to do anything like that to be a "real" duathlete? Not at all. Any duathlon for anyone who does one is a very real experience for him or her. (See chapter 11 for further comments on this subject.) But whatever your limitations are, there are limits to be explored, that is, if you want to explore them.

No. 5, Gradual change leads to permanent changes, will be obvious to any reader who has gotten this far in this book. Slow and steady wins the race to becoming physically fit, to becoming a successful, happy duathlete, to getting to the starting line for your first race or for your fiftieth, and then, most times, crossing the finish line, happily and healthily. As for the race itself, that is of course another matter. But if you try to get to that starting line without putting in the necessary mental and physical training that this book is all about, that is, if you try to "jump right in," the very likely result is going to be pain if not injury, frustration leading to anger, and then to quitting. Not the result you want.

This all leads to the final point, No. 6, Understanding that while we can never be perfect, we can always get better, whether better means faster or longer or simply staying with it over time when you never had the foggiest notion that you would be able to do so. Perfectionism invariably will lead you down the road to failure. Getting better, as long as you define "better" reasonably and rationally for yourself and where you are in your life, will almost invariably lead to continued success, on your own terms.

On Willpower

And yes, there's the old saw, "What you need is will power." Indeed this is one old saw that still cuts. As much as some "experts" on various kinds of health-promoting behavior will tell you that you *don't* need willpower, in my view that is a totally misleading statement. It is designed, certainly with good intentions, to make you think that making the change, whatever it is, is easier than it really is. But change is never easy, although some changes are easier to make than others. In terms of personal health-related behavior change, the term "willpower" means *the conscious mental ability to follow through on plans to make change and to maintain the change once it is made.*

If anyone says that any health-promoting behavior change can be achieved without willpower, they are blowing smoke. You do have to get organized to mobilize your motivation. That takes focus, that takes concentration, that takes commitment. That means engaging your mental capacities to make a change in the way you live your life—nothing more and nothing less. Yes, you do have to have the conscious mental ability to do that. And that, dear reader, is willpower. To get where you want to go, you have to have it. It's as simple, and as complicated, as that.

Final Thought

I hope that you now can see that if you can follow these steps for changing your life to become a duathlete, or if you have done a race or two or three, to become a better organized and healthier duathlete, you can then apply them to making any other personal health-promoting behavior change you want to make. It is in this way that duathlon can come to be at the center of your whole pattern of healthy living.

References

Jonas, S. and E. Phillips. *ACSM's Exercise Is Medicine: A Clinician's Guide to Exercise Prescription*. Philadelphia: Lippincott, Williams and Wilkins, 2009.

Office of Disease Prevention and Health Promotion. *2008 Physical Activity Guidelines for Americans*. Washington, DC: United States Department of Health and Human Services, ODPHP Publication No. U0036, October 2008.

CHAPTER 11

After Crossing the Finish Line: Food for Thought

We have come a long way together in this book. I hope that I have been able to help you organize your thoughts about duathlon racing, set up a training program that works for you, gather your equipment, learn the technical skills you need to learn, find a race or two (or more) to do, get to the starting line ready to go while staying within yourself, and cross that finish line happily and healthily. I hope, too, that you will be set up mentally and physically for a lifetime in the sport, whether you do a race or two or eight to ten a year. In this chapter, I want to share with you some more of my personal experiences in and perspectives on the sport, as well as those of others, that will cast further light on why we do it, what we get out of it, and why some of us at least will stay with it for as long as our legs can carry us.

My First Duathlon

My first duathlon was one of Dan Honig's early Brooklyn Biathlons. It was held on a rainy day in May, 1984, on the old Naval Air Station, Floyd Bennett Field, just off Jamaica Bay (actually just across the Brooklyn/Queens border in Queens, New York City). It was just my third multisport race. I had begun my career in the sport with two triathlons the previous September. Not wanting to wait for the first triathlon in the area in June, I decided to try this then-new variant of multi-sport racing. As noted earlier in the book, Dan had first come up with the "biathlon" idea in order to extend the season at both ends for triathletes in the New York Metropolitan area. And there I was at the starting line, in the rain.

There weren't too many of us way back then, but one of my fellow competitors was a woman with grayish-white hair who looked to be in her fifties. I got to chatting with her. First multisport race? Yes. Running background? No. First race ever, then? Yes. In the rain? Yes. Are you going to finish? Yes I am! And she did. As did I, in an hour and thirty-eight minutes, in the rain. (Yes indeed, as a previous nonathlete, except for skiing, I was elated to find a sport that I could actually not only do but have fun doing. Thus I have kept a record of every single multisport race that I have ever been in since.) Ordinarily, I don't race on rainy days, for reasons of safety and comfort. But the course for that race was absolutely flat, there was no traffic, and on the bike I made very wide and slow turns. I was soaked but oh-so-happy at the finish. And so, I am happy to report to you that I have been doing duathlons for almost as long as I have been doing triathlons, in a ratio of about two du's to every three tri's. Obviously, I have had a great time in both multisport variants over the years. Which brings us to the following question.

What Is a "Real" Duathlete?

In the October 2010 issue of *Inside Triathlon,* one Ms. Katherine Wurzer published a letter that read, in part: "Some time ago, I participated in a sprint-distance triathlon. The race took me a few months to prepare for, was a lot of fun and got me excited about multisport. . . . Here's my problem: [Some say] that I didn't really do a triathlon and that I'm lying whenever I tell people I did, even though I always use the 'sprint-distance' qualifier. [Some say] that only the ironman distance counts as a triathlon. Am I misleading people, including myself, when I say I did a triathlon if the race was only a sprint?"

"Only a sprint," you say. Gee, I wonder what that makes those of us who competed in the Sprint Triathlon National Championships at Cayuga Lake, New York, in 2009 or at Tuscaloosa, Alabama, in 2010? Or those folks who compete in the International Triathlon Union Sprint Triathlon World Championships that have been held every year since 2008? Not "real" triathletes? And then if you are a duathlete, are you not "real" if most of the races you do are at the sprint-distance (one good reason for that being that the overwhelming majority of duathlons, in the United States at least, are at that distance)? Are you a "real" duathlete only if you've done the old Liberty-to-Liberty Biathlon (Jersey City, New Jersey, to Philadelphia, Pennsylvania; see below) or Dan Honig's old Empire State Biathlon (also see below) or the Powerman in Alabama or Zofingen, Switzerland (no, don't look below; I've done neither one. But I did mention them in chapter 1).

Well, it depends how you define "real," I guess. For a while an editorial writer for one of our leading triathlon magazines used to write about triathlon as if doing an ironman was the gold standard, and getting to the Hawaii Ironman at Kona was the diamond/gold standard. Fortunately, that writer stopped doing that. For what does that kind of message, the message delivered to the writer of the letter above, say to those duathletes who will never get to do a Powerman or an intermediate distance Du for that matter? "Forget it. You don't count. Don't think that you have done anything. Don't imagine for an instant that the training you put in, the discipline you exerted during that training, the focus you had on the day of the race, the pride you felt on getting to the starting line and even more so when you crossed the finish line, mean anything." Obviously, wrong message, reflecting some serious problems of self-image in the mind of the sender, reflecting nothing of meaning at all onto the intended recipient(s).

As I write this, I am midway through my twenty-ninth season in multisport racing. I have done more than 85 duathlons and 130 triathlons. It happens that between 1985 and 1994, I was lucky enough to have started five ironman distance triathlons five times and finish three of them. (The other two times I got halfway on the marathon, was not going to make the time limit, and had to drop out.) I have also competed in three long-distance duathlons, finishing one (running out of time on one and being felled by the heat on the other one I didn't finish). They were "real" experiences, I can tell you, and I am very happy that I had the chance to do them. But just as real for me was that very first duathlon, in the rain in 1984, and, for example, my first one of the 2011 season, Dan Honig's March Madness Duathlon (yes, Dan now uses that name for his two-sport races), which I finished in forty-degree weather wearing a ski helmet and a balaclava, and every other duathlon that I have done on warm, sunny days and other types of weather in between.

Why "real?" There is absolutely no absolute standard for "real." If for the person who told the letter writer that the only "real" triathlon is an ironman, all that means is that the only "real" triathlon for him is an ironman. For what does the word "real" really mean? Something that you experience objectively, something that you can see or taste or hear or feel, that has an actual existence for you, not necessarily for anybody else. So whatever the race was, whether it was long, short, or in between; whether it was on a hot, cold, windy, calm, or in-between day; whether it was hilly, flat, or in-between. Was it fun, or even if it weren't fun on a given Sunday, was gutting it out and crossing the finish line *real* for you? Then for you, it was a real race, a real experience.

And actually, on some days if you did the best you could do on that day and happened not to finish, as Dave Scott, one of the greatest triathletes of all time and the first "Ironman" elected to the USAT Hall of Fame, said a long time ago (this favorite and much-used quote of mine is on the frontispiece of the original edition of *Triathloning for Ordinary Mortals*, and the second edition too): "I encourage all . . . triathletes to reach for their goals, whether they be to win or just to try. The trying is everything." Which leads me to Not Finishing.

On Not Finishing

The 1990 Independence Day Liberty-to-Liberty Biathlon (Jersey City, New Jersey, to Philadelphia, Pennsylvania). The day dawned crisp and clear. At 6:00 a.m. the temperature was about sixty degrees Farehenheit, going up to seventy-five. The humidity was low, and there was little wind. A perfect day for long-distance racing. Unfortunately, those were the conditions along the course of the race two days before the event. OK, let's try again. The day dawned sunny, with moderate humidity, the temperature set to peak in the low eighties, with a strong east to northeast wind. An almost perfect day for this race. Although it was a bit warm and humid, we would have close to a tail wind all the way to Philly on the bike. A downwind glide. Personal records for the century (100-mile bike ride) all round. Wow! Unfortunately, those were the conditions two days *after* the event. On the day of the race, July *4th,* 1990, the conditions were quite different.

On that July 4, I first ventured out of the race headquarters hotel, the Newark Airport Radisson, at 6:00 a.m. As a native New Yorker I already knew that we were in for one of those traditional hazy, hot, and humid days of summer. The temperature would go into the high nineties, the humidity into the eighties.

But the worst of it for many of us that day was the wind: never less than twenty mph, with stronger gusts, *from the southwest*. The 100-mile bike segment ran from the Liberty State Park in Jersey City, New Jersey, just across from the Statue of Liberty in New York Harbor, to Independence Plaza in front of Independence Hall, where rests the Liberty Bell, in Philadelphia, Pennsylvania. The bike leg was preceded by a 10-kilometer run in Liberty State Park and followed by another on the streets of Philadelphia. That southwest wind, thus, was right on the nose all the way down the bike course. During the race, I kept waiting for the wind to diminish. It never did.

The shadeless first 10-kilometer run got underway in the Park at about 8:30 a.m. Unlike in most multisport races, in this one the segments did not follow one right after the other. After the run, competitors had to wait around for the bike leg to start. Like most of the other racers, without thinking, I did my waiting around in the sun.

The bike leg itself was divided into two parts: a 32-mile group ride through Staten Island and industrial northern New Jersey and a 68-mile race on through rural New Jersey to the Ben Franklin Bridge and Philadelphia. By the time the group ride got underway at about 10:30 a.m., the temperature had reached about ninety-five degrees with eighty-five percent humidity, being blown right at you by that twenty-mph headwind. I arrived at the southern terminus of the group ride, a small state park in north central New Jersey, feeling okay, but just okay.

Again, competitors had to wait for the start of the next segment. Again I made the mistake of standing around in the sun, instead of seeking some shade. The start for the bike race was staggered, in order of finish in the first run, the first finishers going off first on the bike. Thus I was one of the last to get underway on the bike. By now I had been in the sun, as well as the hot atmosphere, for a long time.

The first few miles of the bike course were uphill. By mile 45 (total, just 13 miles into the 68-mile race portion) I was not feeling too well. By the 52-mile mark I was last in the bike. By mile 55, my helmet seemed to be shrinking, I was getting nauseated, and a pedal cadence of anything over sixty-five turns per minute (that's rather slow) was impossible. Going downhill, into that wind, I was making a mere 12 miles per hour, while my stomach was slowly making its way toward my mouth. This activity was getting distinctly unhealthy.

And so, I stopped, and got into the shade, too. Fortunately for me, one of the vans assigned to pick up drop-outs (with an accompanying truck to pick up their bikes) came along a few minutes later. Shortly thereafter I was sitting down in air-conditioned comfort. (About 50 percent of the field eventually called it quits that day, one woman only 4 miles from the finish.) On that day, I think that unless extremely fit, you were smart if you recognized your limitations, decided not to explore your limits further, and dropped out. A number of people stayed on the course too long and were taken to the hospital with dehydration or worse. My thoughts? There's always another race, and duathlon is nothing to get sick over.

A number of my van compatriots said that they felt guilty about not finishing. *Guilty?* I thought. Guilty for what? Protecting their health? Recognizing their fatigue? Realizing that their level of training just didn't equip them to deal with such extreme conditions? Disappointed? Yes. A bit down? Sure. Embarrassed in front of friends to whom they might have prematurely boasted a bit? Maybe. But guilty? They had done nothing either immoral or illegal. They had gone as far as they could in the heat, and those in the van had stopped before they got heatstroke. Nothing to feel guilty about.

When I got to Philadelphia, someone asked me how I did. I responded: "I had a great day. I did a 10-kilometer run in the blazing heat and rode 55 really hot miles into a ferocious headwind. Where's the food?" What's the lesson here? Not finishing in itself is not a bad thing. Protecting your health and recognizing that you are simply incapable of reaching a set goal that day are perfectly valid reasons for stopping, and that's a good thing. It's how you react to that event that produces the good, or bad, feelings. And remember. There's always another race.

Which leads me to "On Finishing Last."

On Finishing Last

Do you know why it's better to finish last than sixth from last? Because when you're last everyone knows who you are. When you're sixth from last you're completely anonymous. Finishing my first ironman triathlon, the 1985 Cape Cod Endurance, I was last. But with a couple of miles to go I knew that I was going to beat the seventeen-hour time limit. Actually, I was rolling up the course. When I passed a particular volunteers' station, they were free to pack up and pack it in. But numbers of them did not do the latter. In fact they proceeded to the finish line to await my arrival. As I made the turn onto the last straightaway (and I get goose bumps still as I write this), there were many dozens of them standing there cheering—for me! The theme from *Chariots of Fire* was playing over the loudspeakers. I sprinted the last 200 yards at the end of a seventeen-hour day. Oh what a feeling, with me to this day and beyond.

Then there was the Kaaterskill Spring Rush Prelude (run-ski-bike-run), held at Ski Windham in upper New York State, April, 1998. I was second in my age group but the last finisher, twenty minutes behind the next one in front of me. This time, a group of volunteers (I had once again rolled up the course) came out and put up a tape for me to break as I crossed the finish line. Another unforgettable experience.

Finally, there was Dan Honig's Empire State Biathlon, a 6-mile run, 45-mile bike, plus 6-mile run held in Harriman State Park, New York, in June, 1990. I was twice the age of the next youngest competitor in the race. But I finished, two hours behind the next racer in front of me. And Dan held the finish line open for me. That my dad and step-mom, just a bit older then than I am now, were there to see me make it made it even more special. So, finishing last, just like everything else in multisport racing, is what you make of it.

OK, so even though I've got a bunch of first, second, and third place age-group finish plaques (mainly, as noted, due to the rather modest size of my age group in my region, starting for me at about age sixty), in most of my races I am in the back of the pack pretty much from the get-go.

Which leads us to my . . .

Top Ten Back-of-the-Pack Happenings

1. **"It's easy to find your bike after the first run."** Since most everyone else has come and gone through the first transition by the time I get there, it is indeed easy for me

to find my bike after the first run. And there are very few people to trip over or get in your way as you make your way to the bike exit. This is a definite advantage.

2. **"Aid-station volunteers are saying, 'You can make it' rather than 'Looking good.'"** Actually, some volunteers do say, "Looking good" rather than, "You can make it" or its alternate, "Hang in there." However, most of the time, especially on the second run, I know that those who call out "Looking good!" are either liars or just trying to be kind or need to make a visit to the optometrist. My usual response is, "Appearances can be deceiving."

3. **"Spectators offer you a ride in their car, and you seriously entertain the offer."** That's never happened to me, but there have been a few times when I wish it had.

4. **"It's really difficult to find a place to park your bike before you start the second run."** This is the opposite of No. 1. This is where prerace bike-rack planning and management become very important. First, do try to memorize where your bike-rack spot is. Much time can be wasted hunting around for it, especially in a crowded transition area. Second, try to get to the race early enough so that you can get a spot at one end of your assigned rack or the other, put your bike as close to that end as you can, and then place your stuff on the ground on the inside of your bike as it stands on the rack. Doing this will make it more difficult for anyone else arriving ahead of you to impinge upon your space.

5. **"The volunteers and course marshals are busy working on their tans, instead of watching you."** This may happen at some races, but not in any of the ones that I've done over the years. I generally find volunteers very attentive and usually very encouraging, especially to those of us at the back-of-the-pack. In fact, I try to say something like, "Thanks for being here" to both volunteers and police as I ride by.

6. **"The massage table towels are dirty and soiled."** I've never gone for a massage after a race. I usually don't go fast enough to hurt enough to need it, or alternatively I get in so late that the massage folks have already gone home.

7. **"You begin thanking the aid-station volunteers for staying out on the course for so long."** As noted above, I have had this experience on more than one race. Not only is it a nice gesture on your part, but if you are one of the last persons out there, thanking the volunteers as you pass will increase the chances that they will be motivated to go to the finish line to cheer you in when you finally arrive.

8. **"The fast athletes have finished the race before you even start the second run."** As I have gotten older and slower, I find it hard to remember when this did *not* happen.

9. **"The only place you're not sunburned is where your limbs are marked with your race number."** Since I am fairly dark-skinned, especially during the summer, I can't say that I've experienced this one. But it might be fun to

still be wearing your race number after having taken five showers.

10. **"That old guy riding the Schwinn with a kickstand is trying to draft you."** Wrong. *You* are trying to draft that old guy riding the Schwinn with the kickstand. Or, you *are* that old guy, or gal, riding the Schwinn with the kickstand. Actually, one of the nice things about being in the back of the pack is that most everybody else back there is riding a bike like mine (not a Schwinn with a kickstand, however), one that the person-in-the-street can recognize as a bike that he or she might actually go for a ride on. There's a certain comfort in that, for me anyhow.

Let me conclude by adding my eleventh back-of-the-pack thought: "It's better to be at the back of the pack than not be in the race at all." Which leads me, for no particular reason, to my next subject.

Sex and Duathlon

Charles Dillon "Casey" Stengel was a legendary figure in baseball in the last century, first as a pretty good player and then as one of the greatest managers of all time. If you are not old enough to recognize the name, "you could look it up" (which happened to be one of Casey's favorite sayings). As a manager, for dealing with the press (and sometimes with his ballplayers as well), he invented a variation of the English language known as "Stengelese," a forerunner of the better-known version popularized by Yogi Berra. It was designed, if it were designed, to force listeners to puzzle endlessly over exactly what he meant by what he was saying, for example, "I've always heard it couldn't be done, but sometimes it don't always work."

But he could also be quite straightforward. This brings us straightforwardly to sex and sports. Casey was once asked if he thought that having sex the night before a big game sapped a player's energy. He replied that he wasn't concerned about the energy players might spend in having sex, but rather the energy they might expend in getting it. And so if you are thinking about having sex the night before a duathlon, this concern of Casey's is something to bear in mind.

How about this question? Does duathloning, especially in the Masters' age groups, do anything for one's sex life? Frankly, who knows? Masters duathletes may be multisport athletes because they are sexier, or they may become sexier because they are multisport athletes. Someday, someone might do a survey on that matter. Then, if the results were to be published, we could say, in Casey Stengel's immortal words, "you could look it up."

As you could look up Jeff Matlow, a writer, illustrator/cartoonist, triathlete, who publishes regularly in *USAT Magazine* and elsewhere. His Tao of Triathlon (which I have modified slightly, only in the wording, not the meaning, to make it the Tao of Duathlon) appeared in the Spring 2011 issue of the magazine, and is used with his permission and that of our editor, Jayme Ramson, and may not be reprinted without Jeff's permission.

Jeff Matlow (Slightly Modified by Yours Truly): The Tao of Duathlon

Create a racing plan and stick with your plan.

Inevitably, things will happen that won't allow you to stick with your plan.

In case of No. 2, make believe Plan B is your plan. Stick with that one.

No matter how bad and irreparable things may seem, stay the course. It will all eventually get good again.

Every once in a while say something encouraging to another racer. It'll make both of you feel better and the sound of your voice will remind you that you're still alive.

Don't try anything new on race day. Unless it's got the words "chicken" and "soup" in it.

No matter how hard it seems, you had much harder training days.

Before you get to the starting line, make sure you know the reason you are racing duathlon. Write it down; remember it. When things don't go as planned, this will be your source of hope. As Nietzsche's duathlete second cousin once said, "he who has a why to race a duathlon can bear with almost any how."

Come up with a motivating mantra. The right mantra can be your best friend. "Slow is smooth, smooth is fast."

"Train hard; race easy." "Be here now." Whatever it is, you'll be surprised how well a few simple words will keep you focused and on track.

Be here now (see, the mantra works already). Don't worry about what is behind you, and stop your mind from thinking about what lies ahead. All you can affect is right here, right now. It is one pedal, one step. And you just need to focus on doing that one thing to the absolute best of your ability and keep repeating it until they tell you to stop.

Figure out what you need to eat and drink months before you get to the starting line. All the training in the world will add up to a load of bull puckey if you don't pay attention to your body.

Don't wear yourself out on the first run. For most of us, a duathlon doesn't really begin until halfway through the second run anyway. If you pace yourself well, you'll be zipping by people during those last miles while all the folks that left it all on the bike course will be gasping for energy. Try not to kick them in the face as you run them over; that's just plain rude.

Don't worry; be happy. As Yogi Berra's duathlete neighbor's uncle once said, racing a duathlon is 90 percent mental; the other half is physical. [Neither of them knew Bob Roses; see chapter 3.] Maintaining a calm, positive attitude throughout the day is often the difference between a good race and a really crappy one.

Remind yourself regularly that you are racing a duathlon, and you're darn lucky to have the ability and means to do this. Relish the experience. Enjoy the day. The miracle isn't that you will finish and you will. The miracle is that you had the courage to start.

Getting Started Later in Life: The Drs. Sheehan and Ogilvie

I had first heard of the late Dr. George Sheehan, the original "Guru of Running," back in the 1970s, some years before I started running myself. George was the first running writer to explore the spiritual side of the sport, and he hit a responsive chord among the many folks who were taking up the sport for the first time. George had begun running when he was forty-five or so, about the same age as I was when I took up the sport about twenty years after he did. But one big difference between George and me was that he was fast. He loved to race, did it with great frequency, and consistently won in his age group. And to him, running was the distance sport. Not swimming, not biking.

When back in 1986 I sent him a copy of *Triathloning for Ordinary Mortals,* his comment was along the lines that the sport was cobbled together; it was not real, not pure, like running. But one of George's most admirable characteristics was the ability to look at himself, to grow, to change. And so, when an illness slowed down his running somewhat, George tried biking and found that he liked it. He had been a swimmer in his youth and lived near the New Jersey shore. Obviously, for an adventuresome sort like George, triathlon was not far behind. In his late sixties, he took it up with his customary verve. Soon he became a proponent of the sport.

And then there was my friend and colleague, Dr. Charles Ogilvie, professor of the history of medicine at the Texas College of Osteopathic Medicine in Fort Worth and a former radiologist, who, in my early days in the sport, helped to turn me into a runner. Overweight as an adult, but a former college sprinter, Charlie first took up distance running at age fifty-eight. By the time he was sixty he weighed 170 pounds. He was doing marathons in just over three hours, blowing away most everyone else in his age group and many younger than him as well. Charlie celebrated his sixty-fifth year by doing ten marathons, all in the low three-hour range. But when Charlie turned sixty-eight, he decided that it was time to take up something new. He turned to triathlon and he became pretty fast at that too. It turned out, however, that his mother, still living well into her nineties, was concerned. "Charles," she one day said to him, "do you really think that it is safe for a man of your age to be riding a bicycle on the public roads?"

Let me conclude this chapter with some of the thought of Dr. Sheehan. A very wise man was he, about racing, about life, and about being. I would like to share some of that thought with you as you enter on the life pathway of becoming and being a duathlete.

The Thought of George Sheehan

George's next-to-last book, *Personal Best*, is a guide to living the healthy life in body, mind, and spirit. But this book does not present my kind of left-brain, orderly (compulsive to some) approach. My kind of plan, of course, is more on the order of, "This is the topic we are addressing, this is the problem, this is the solution, and this is how to implement it." (Yes, that's right—like the approach I take in this book). George's plan has instead the right-brain kind of plan he was so comfortable with. (I'm working on it; I'm working on it!)

The essence of George Sheehan was that even when a life experience was not a happy one—getting cancer, losing a loving relationship—he thought, he felt, and he could, if he put his mind to it, become a better person for it. George never lost his love of life, his zest for it, and his ability to learn from it, even as he was in the last stages of his own life. Like the good, competitive duathlete, and Satchel Paige, he never looked back, but always ahead.

Personal Best begins with life and ends with death. Being George Sheehan, our author managed to deal with both in an upbeat, optimistic fashion. I cannot do justice to George's prose by trying to describe it. Rather, I will share with you a few of my favorite quotes from the book.

On life: "The normal life was one of continual expansion." "Life is not a skill sport. . . . It is a game that anyone can play and play well." "The diligent use of our allotted life span is the secret of the successful life."

On death: "Death makes the everyday magical, the ordinary unique, the commonplace one-of-a-kind." "Once I accept death, I center on the present." "To have a death worth dying, you must have a life worth living."

In between life and death, George talked about motivation, setting goals, running for the mind, the true meaning of racing, happiness, sadness, love, aloneness, relationships, the mind and healthy aging, and being healthy. Exquisite thoughts are to be found on almost every page. Let me just share a few more of them with you.

On motivation: "No motivation can live where faith and courage are absent." On goal setting: "My end is not simple happiness. My need, drive, and desire is to achieve my full and complete self." On health: "Health makes for the happy pursuit of happiness and gives us a longer time to do it." On racing: "It's the race that challenges me, not the finish line." On exercise and health: "The simplest way to preserve health is to exercise." On running and the mind: "So where do you find the life of the mind? Within yourself, the self that is nurtured and freed by running." And finally, on happiness: "Happiness we receive from ourselves is greater than that we receive from our surroundings."

George Sheehan died of prostate cancer on November 1, 1993. There will never be another like him. He had a unique gift: the ability to communicate with virtually everyone, expressing thoughts that reflect the center of man's exis-tence. We are all the better for having had George Sheehan, who happened to become a multisport racer late in life, in our midst.

CHAPTER 12

Additional Resources

At the time of publication of this book, there were no other modern books solely devoted to duathlon. Two had been published in the 1990s, but they were long out of date. However, there are two reasons that you might be interested in finding out about resources other than this book. First, you might be interested in going faster as a duathlete, something we don't deal with in this book. There are numbers of triathlon books which do deal with that subject and of course the running and cycling sections in these books are applicable to going fast in duathlon as well as triathlon.

One that I like to recommend is a book that I had a hand in, *Championship Triathlon Training: Advanced Training for Peak Performance,* (George Dallam, Ph.D., and yours truly, Champaign, IL: Human Kinetics, 2008). George is a good friend and also one of the top multisport coaches in the country. Among his clients was Hunter Kemper, the only man to have been on all three US Olympic Triathlon Teams to date (2011). It's George's book. I helped out with a few of the ideas and a good deal of the editing. Velo Press also has a couple of titles that are sport-specific: *The Triathlete's Guide to Bike Training* and *The Triathlete's Guide to Run Training*. They are of course as easily applicable to duathlon as they are to triathlon. Authors in the Velo stable whom I know personally and know to produce high-quality work are Joe Friel and Gale Bernhardt. Again, the run and bike sections of their books are as applicable to duathlon as to triathlon.

The second reason you may be interested in other resources is that perhaps you may want to add triathloning to your multisport quiver someday. For getting started, I must say that I do like two books of mine. *Triathloning for Ordinary Mortals* (New York: WW Norton, 1986; 2nd ed., 2006) was the first book for beginners and recreational triathletes on the sport. As of 2011 it has sold over forty-six thousand copies. Then there is my 2011 book, *101 Ideas and Insights for Triathletes and Duathletes,* (Monterey, CA: Healthy Learning/Coaches Choice). Like this book and *Triathloning for Ordinary Mortals, 101 Ideas* is about getting started and staying with it at the recreational level. Joe Friel and Gale Bernhardt both have books for beginners as well, perhaps a little more oriented to performance as an eventual goal than mine are.

As far as periodicals are concerned, there are three at the national level. *USA Triathlon Magazine* is a quarterly put out by the organization for its members. (Full disclosure: I write a regular column for it under the title "Ordinary Mortals®: Talking Triathlon with Steve Jonas.") There are two national magazines published by the same company, Competitor Group (http://competitorgroup.com/). *Triathlete* is a monthly with up-to-the-minute race information, product reviews, and training advice. *Inside Triathlon*, a bi-monthly, is for the most part oriented to long-form feature articles about the sport and the people in it who make it go.

Websites abound. The only one that focuses primarily on duathlon is www.dualthlon.com, edited and published by one of this book's endorsers, Eric Schwartz. It also covers triathlon to a certain extent. USA Triathlon's website is www.usa triathlon.org (which from now on will be featuring duathlon as well as triathlon and the other forms of multisport racing). You can find out just about everything here, from what USAT is and how to join, to sport news, resources, event schedules, rules, and the programs for training and certifying coaches and race directors. Another major website is www.active .com, which covers many sports (go to the Endurance button for multisport); to go directly to multi-sport on Active.com, for schedules, news, and training tips visit www.active.com/ triathlon/Newsletters/. Mainly focused on multisport racing, www.slowtwitch.com has product reviews, race reports, personal interviews, and some sport gossip. *Triathlete* magazine also has a broad-coverage website at http://triathlon.competitor.com/.

As I noted at the end of chapter 4, there are a number of websites that publish race calendars. You can find them, for example (as of 2011), at www.trifind.com/, www.trifind.net/, www.race360.com/triathlon/races/, www.calendar.slowtwitch .com/, www.lin-mark.com/, and www.beginnertriathlete.com. *Triathlete* magazine (http://triathlon.competitor.com/) periodically publishes race calendars and/or information about upcoming races. You can find a national list of local triathlon/ duathlon clubs put together by USA Triathlon at their website, www.usatriathlon.org/resources/for-clubs/find-a-club.

So. You've got your advice on training, racing, technique, equipment, duathlon as part of a healthy lifestyle and philosophy of life, and additional resources. Now all you need to do is make up your mind to go out there and Du it.

Index

About the Author

Steven Jonas, MD, MPH, is also the author of *The Essential Triathlete* (Lyons Press), *Championship Triathlon Training* with top triathlon coach George Dallam, Ph.D., and *101 Ideas and Insights for Triathletes and Duathletes*. He has written regular columns on triathlons for more than twenty years. In addition to being a veteran multisport racer, he was a member of the National Coaching Commission of USA Triathlon (2000–2002). He is professor of preventive medicine at the School of Medicine, and professor, Graduate Program in Public Health at Stony Brook University. He received his MD from the Harvard Medical School, his MPH from the Yale School of Medicine, and his MS in health management from New York University. He is board certified in preventive medicine, and is a fellow of the New York Academy of Sciences (elected), the American College of Preventive Medicine, the American Public Health Association, the New York Academy of Medicine, and the Royal Society of Medicine (UK). He lives in Port Jefferson, New York.

He is married to Mrs. Chezna Newman of New York City, has two children of his own, Jacob Henry Jonas and Lillian Jonas Wain, two grandchildren, Nathan Harold Wain and Adam Jonas Wain, and a stepson, Mark Newman.